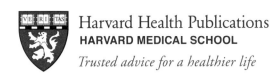

Dear Reader,

All your life, your skin has been making a first impression for you. It can reveal whether you're hot or cold, tired or rested, sick or healthy. As you age, your skin changes in response to the elements that assail it, particularly the sun. On the inside, you may feel as good as ever, but on the outside, your skin may send a different message. Over the years, everyday stresses and exposures alter your skin's tone, texture, and contour.

To some extent, your genes determine how well your skin stands the test of time. But environmental factors, such as sun exposure, play a big role as well, affecting not just your skin's appearance, but also your risk of skin cancer. Each year, physicians diagnose more than five million cases of two highly curable forms of skin cancer—basal cell carcinoma and squamous cell carcinoma. But for nearly 77,000 people, the diagnosis will be melanoma, a potentially deadly form of skin cancer. That's why it's so important to minimize your exposure to ultraviolet radiation. The World Health Organization places people who use ultraviolet tanning beds in its highest cancer risk category. If it's vitamin D you're after, tanning beds are not a good choice, but spending a very short time in the sun is safe for most people.

When it comes to skin treatments, there's lots of good news in therapies for medical conditions as well as cosmetic concerns. But it's important to choose your treatments with care and to check and double-check the reputation and accreditation of clinicians performing invasive skin procedures. The market for skin treatments is skyrocketing: Americans spend an estimated $5 billion each year on anti-aging skin care products, and the number of cosmetic procedures to improve the skin's appearance has increased to more than 16 million annually in the United States, with nonsurgical procedures making up 14 million of the total.

This report is intended to help you sort through your options by providing information based on scientific research and my own experience as a physician. You'll find authoritative information about common and age-related skin conditions. A detailed section on cosmetic techniques ranging from laser resurfacing to cosmetic fillers can help you decide whether such procedures might be right for you. These are highly personal decisions. Whatever choices you make, you have more options today than ever before.

Sincerely,

Kenneth A. Arndt, M.D.

Kenneth A. Arndt, M.D.
Medical Editor

Editor's note: Dr. Arndt reports owning stock in PhotoMedex, which makes lasers for treating psoriasis and vitiligo.

Skin: The basics

Although most people seldom stop to appreciate their skin, it's much more than a simple covering. It is the body's largest organ—it weighs about nine pounds—and it carries out a number of functions that help maintain health.

Your skin is actually a complex fabric of tissues working together to protect you in multiple ways. On the most obvious level, it forms a defensive barrier, protecting your inner organs from foreign invaders such as bacteria and viruses. But it is not just a passive wall: in the outermost layer of skin, cells called Langerhans cells actively ward off infections, forming the front-line defenses of the immune system.

Your skin is also a sensory organ. Nerve endings on its surface pick up and relay information about the surrounding environment to your brain. Your brain then translates these nerve impulses into the sensations of heat and cold, as well as touch, pressure, and pain. If you touch a scalding pot, for example, the warning signals cause you to pull back in an instant, before further harm is done. Or, if the room is too hot or too cold, these sensations tell you to turn on the fan or put on a sweater. But your skin actively contributes to temperature control, too. When you're hot, it helps cool you down by sweating and dilating its blood vessels. When you're cold, those blood vessels constrict to conserve heat deep inside your body.

Finally, the skin is also a manufacturing plant, using the sun's energy to make vitamin D, which is essential to many body functions.

Skin layers, explained

To carry out all these functions, the skin relies on the specialized structures in its three layers—the epidermis, the dermis, and the subcutaneous layer, sometimes called the hypodermis or fat layer (see Figure 1).

The outermost layer

The epidermis—the outermost layer of the skin—is a protective, physical barrier, about as thick as a piece of

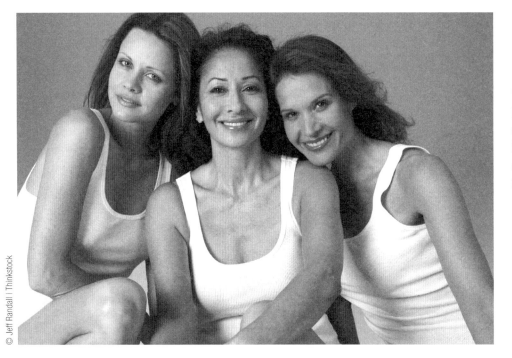

Your skin is your body's largest organ, weighing about nine pounds, and it carries out a number of functions that help you maintain your health.

paper. The very top portion of the epidermis is known as the stratum corneum. It's composed of cells called keratinocytes that produce a tough protein called keratin, forming a flexible outer shield. As younger cells from the lower part of the epidermis rise to the surface from below, the older cells die and are rubbed off or fall off. This continuous cycle completely renews the skin surface about once a month.

The epidermis plays a key role in protecting you from the sun's radiation. In particular, pigmented cells called melanocytes are located at the bottom of the epidermis. These cells produce the melanin, or pigment, that colors skin and helps protect against ultraviolet radiation. When exposed to sunlight, the melanocytes churn out more melanin, and the skin darkens to help shield against further damage. If the melanocytes become cancerous, the condition is termed melanoma.

The middle layer

The dermis lies directly beneath the epidermis. It is a thicker layer that contains collagen, blood and lymph vessels, nerves, hair follicles, and glands that produce sweat and oil. Blood vessels in the dermis expand or contract to maintain a constant body temperature. White blood cells patrol the dermis to fight infectious microbes that manage to break through the epidermis. Cells called fibroblasts secrete collagen, which gives the skin its strength and firmness. Elastin fibers made of protein in the dermis give skin its elasticity.

The deepest layer

The subcutaneous tissue (hypodermis), which consists of connective tissue and fat, lies between the dermis and underlying muscles or bones. It, too, contains blood vessels and infection-fighting white blood cells, but not to the same extent as in the dermis. Fat in the subcutaneous layer stores nutrients and insulates and cushions muscles and bones.

Nails and hair

Your nails are skin, too. They're a thickened, hardened form of epidermis. Nail cells originate from the base of the nail bed. They die quickly, but unlike the keratinocytes, they aren't sloughed off. They're also composed of a much stronger form of keratin. Thus, a nail is simply a sheet of keratin like the topmost layer of skin, but much harder and thicker. By contrast, hair is a thin fiber made of many overlapping layers of keratin, which is produced in the hair follicle. ♥

Figure 1: An inside look at skin

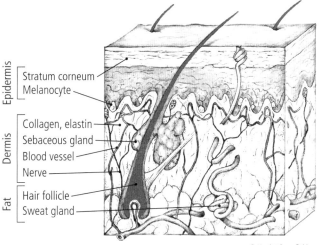

Epidermis
— Stratum corneum
— Melanocyte

Dermis
— Collagen, elastin
— Sebaceous gland
— Blood vessel
— Nerve

Fat
— Hair follicle
— Sweat gland

© Harriet Greenfield

Skin is more than just a cosmetic covering for the body. It forms a protective physical barrier against germs and toxins. Its blood vessels and sweat glands regulate body temperature. Its immune cells ward off infection. Tiny nerve cells detect pressure and temperature, and other skin cells manufacture vitamin D.

Skin and the aging process

It seems a paradox: if the top layer of skin is replaced about once a month, why does skin age? There are multiple reasons, which are explained in this chapter.

Chronological aging

Time takes its toll. As the years go by, skin undergoes a number of biochemical changes. For one, epidermal cells don't slough off as easily, and the supportive fibers of collagen and elastin in the dermis break down. The deterioration of collagen and elastin and the pull of gravity can result in some of the classic signs of aging skin: fine lines around the eyes, deepened expression lines at the corners of the mouth and across the forehead, and sagging skin. The nails usually become more brittle, and hair may begin to thin.

Age-related bone loss in the skull also affects your appearance. Many people develop nasolabial folds (sometimes called smile lines), which are lines from each side of the nose to the corners of the mouth, as the result of underlying changes in their facial bones, not drooping skin per se. The same is true for melomental folds (marionette lines), which run from the corners of the mouth to the chin.

But there are other changes in the skin as well. With aging, skin doesn't retain as much moisture as it once did. Its ability to fight infection, feel sensations, and regulate body temperature also diminishes. And over several decades of sending instructions for new cell production, the DNA in skin cells can become damaged and allow cells to grow out of control, with skin cancer as the result.

Part of the aging process is genetic. Just as your genetic makeup determines your eye color and whether your hair is curly or straight, genes also play a role in determining whether your skin retains a firm texture into your 60s and 70s, or begins to wrinkle and sag during your 40s. The breakdown of collagen and elastin that leads to droopy, lax skin occurs at different rates in different people.

Photoaging

The single biggest cause of damage to your skin as you age is not aging itself—it's sun exposure. This damage is called photoaging, and people spend billions of dollars annually to counteract its effects. Over the years, sun exposure causes fine and coarse wrinkles; baggy skin with a yellow, leathery appearance; and dry, scaly skin. It also increases the risk for skin cancer. Because

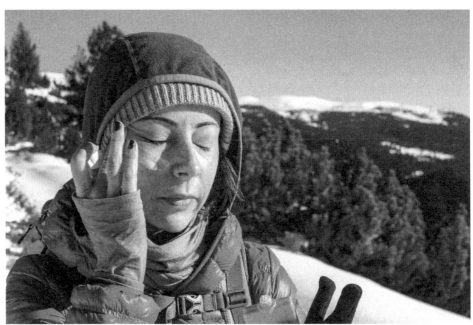

Even in winter, it pays to protect your skin from ultraviolet light. Over the years, excess sun exposure causes lines, wrinkles, and leathery skin, and increases your risk of skin cancer.

© Stuny | Thinkstock

sun exposure diminishes collagen, which supports a network of blood vessels, photoaging can also cause skin to bruise more easily.

You can readily distinguish the effects of photoaging from those of chronological aging by performing this simple test. Look at the lines and pigmentation of the skin on your face and the backs of your hands and feel the skin's texture. Now do the same on a part of your body that hasn't received much sun exposure over the years, such as your lower abdomen or buttocks. The difference can be dramatic, especially if you've been a sun worshipper throughout your life.

The role of ultraviolet light

Skin damage from sun exposure is caused by ultraviolet (UV) radiation, but not all of the sun's UV rays have the same effects. Some wavelengths of UV radiation penetrate the skin more deeply than others (see Figure 2). Realizing this difference has prompted researchers to question whether some types of UV rays mainly cause wrinkles and brown spots (sometimes called "age spots" or "liver spots"), while others speed the development of skin cancer.

The wavelengths of UV radiation fall between those of visible light and x-rays. The sun's UV radiation comes in three main wavelengths.

UVC. This wavelength is the shortest of the three. It also has the highest energy level and is capable of destroying the skin, but these rays are usually absorbed in the atmosphere by the ozone layer before they reach the earth's surface. In the 1970s, concerns about holes in the ozone layer led to global bans of ozone-depleting chemicals, and today the ozone layer appears to be repairing itself.

UVB. These rays are slightly longer and lower in energy than UVC rays, so they're less damaging to skin, but you're exposed to more of them. They make up around 5% of the ultraviolet radiation that reaches the earth's surface. UVB rays penetrate the epidermis, and the immediate result of their damage is a sunburn. Over time, cumulative exposure to UVB leads to photoaging lines and wrinkles. Experts also gen-

Figure 2: Three wavelengths of skin damage

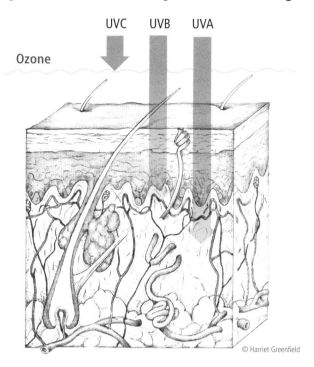

© Harriet Greenfield

Three wavelengths of ultraviolet (UV) light come from the sun. UVA is the longest wavelength and penetrates most deeply. UVB is the next longest. UVC, the shortest wavelength, is normally blocked by the atmosphere's ozone layer. All UV rays can cause damage to the skin.

erally believe that the more often you've been sunburned, the more likely you are to develop melanoma. Research suggests that UVB rays cause a distinctive genetic mutation that permits unabated cell growth, giving rise to cancer. In fact, more than 90% of squamous cell cancers have this specific mutation.

UVA. The rays with the longest range of wavelengths, called UVA, also play a role in photoaging and in the development of skin cancer. About 95% of the UV radiation that reaches the earth's surface is UVA. Because of their longer wavelength, these rays penetrate more deeply into the dermis, damaging deep connective tissue and leading to the appearance of leathery skin. Only about 10% of UVB rays reach the dermis, but researchers believe that 50% of UVA rays do so. ▼

Common skin conditions

Throughout your life, chances are good that you'll experience one or more problems that affect your skin. These afflictions range from unsightly but generally harmless conditions (such as rosacea and warts) to more serious problems, such as psoriasis and shingles. In addition, a small number of people are born with birthmarks, skin discolorations that are nearly always harmless (see Table 1).

This chapter contains brief descriptions of some of the most common skin problems, along with advice about how to prevent, treat, and manage them.

Adult acne

Although most common during the teenage years, acne may also appear for the first time in midlife or worsen then. Acne results from inflammation around the hair follicles and oil-producing sebaceous glands of the skin. Hormones known as androgens (the so-called male hormones), which increase during puberty in both males and females, contribute to acne. Hormonal fluctuations associated with menstruation and menopause make women more susceptible.

Table 1: From café au lait to strawberries: Common birthmarks

Birthmarks, which are painless skin discolorations, show up at birth or soon after and come in a range of shapes, sizes, and colors. They are caused by extra pigment in the skin or blood vessels that don't form correctly.

TYPE	APPEARANCE	USUAL LOCATION	PROGNOSIS AND TREATMENT
Congenital mole (nevus)	Brown; shape and size vary.	Anywhere on body.	Persists throughout life; no treatment needed. However, very large nevi pose a higher risk of melanoma, so people with these need to follow them carefully.
Café-au-lait spot	Light to chocolate brown, smooth, oval.	Torso, buttocks, legs.	Persists throughout life. Can be treated with lasers but with variable success.
Mongolian spot	Smooth, blue or blue-gray, often uneven in shape.	Lower back and buttocks; more common in Asian and black children.	Usually fades within first year of life; can be covered with opaque creams such as Dermablend or Covermark.
Salmon patch (nevus simplex)	Flat patch of pink or red skin, often small, with poorly defined borders; seen in up to one in three newborns.	Nape of the neck ("stork bite"), between the eyebrows ("angel's kiss"), or on the eyelids.	Usually fades within first year of life.
Strawberry hemangioma	Raised blue, red, or purple; soft; compressible with well-defined borders; shape and size vary; seen in up to 3% of newborns.	Face, scalp, chest, or back; may appear at age 1–2 months. May extend deeper than the skin and in rare cases interfere with vital organs.	Often grows from ages 6 to 12 months, then shrinks and disappears by 9 years of age. Deeper or larger lesions (which sometimes interfere with a vital organ) may be treated with topical, oral, or injected steroids or other medications; laser therapy; or surgery.
Port-wine stain (nevus flammeus)	Flat patch of purple or dark red skin, often large, with well-defined borders; occurs in less than 1% of infants.	One side of the face or neck.	May darken or thicken and develop tiny bumps as the person ages. Can be covered with opaque creams such as Dermablend or Covermark; can also be treated with laser therapy.

▶ Symptoms of adult acne

✔ Whiteheads (closed, plugged oil glands)

✔ Blackheads (open, plugged oil glands)

✔ Pustules (swollen red bumps), sometimes filled with pus

Treating adult acne

A number of treatments are available to clear up acne, including some that you apply to your skin and others you take in pill form.

First-line topical treatments typically fall into one of these two categories:

Salicylic acid washes. These formulas loosen dead skin cells and help dislodge plugs from pore openings, seen as whiteheads and blackheads. Salicylic acid washes are available in over-the-counter and prescription formulations, but the prescription versions aren't any stronger.

Benzoyl peroxide gels, lotions, and washes. These products fight bacterial growth and may help clear blocked pores. They are available in over-the-counter and prescription versions. They can induce side effects such as dry and peeling skin if the formulation is too strong or is used excessively, or if a person has very sensitive skin.

For more active or serious cases, doctors can prescribe any of the following:

Topical retinoids. Available as creams, gels, or liquids, these drugs help clear the skin of plugged follicles by increasing the turnover of skin cells. The most common one, tretinoin (Retin-A, generic), may cause skin irritation. Other topical retinoids include adapalene (Differin), which is the first topical retinoid available over the counter (in a 0.1% formulation, although there is also a 0.3% gel available by prescription), and tazarotene (Tazorac). To avoid side effects such as drying, peeling, and redness, begin by using retinoids twice a week at night and gradually move up to every-other-night or nightly use. Because these medications may increase the skin's sensitivity to sunlight, while you are using them always be sure to apply sunscreen during the day.

Oral retinoid. Isotretinoin (Amnesteem, Claravis, others) is used to treat chronic, severe, or disfiguring acne. Because this medication has been associated with serious side effects, including severe birth defects and possibly inflammatory bowel disease, depression, and suicidal thoughts, people taking this drug must be registered in a national database and undergo careful monthly monitoring by a dermatologist.

Antibiotics. Certain antibiotics (available as creams, gels, lotions, or combination products) combined with other compounds can be applied directly to the skin to reduce the growth of acne-causing bacteria. Examples include erythromycin plus benzoyl peroxide (Benzamycin); clindamycin plus benzoyl peroxide (Duac, others); sulfacetamide plus sulfur (Plexion TS, others); and dapsone (Aczone). Serious cases are sometimes treated with oral antibiotics, such as doxycycline and minocycline, as well.

Hormonal therapies. Some birth control pills lower androgen levels and help clear up acne in women; these include formulations that contain ethinyl estradiol and norgestimate (Ortho-Cyclen, Ortho Tri-Cyclen, generic) and ethinyl estradiol and drospirenone (Beyasz, Safyral, Yasmin, Yaz, generic). The latter combination is more effective at treating acne than the norgestimate pills, but this benefit must be balanced with its greater potential for causing a blood clot in a vein (called a venous thromboembolism). Spironolactone (Aldactone, generic) is another hormonal medication that can be used in women to supplement the effects of birth control pills or other acne medications; it is particularly helpful to women who experience hormonal flares of their acne. The drug is FDA-approved to treat high blood pressure, but it has also been found to block the effects of androgens on the sebaceous glands and is used "off-label" to manage acne.

Laser and light therapies. These may one day play a role in treating adult acne, but so far, there is little good research to support their use.

Athlete's foot (tinea pedis)

Athlete's foot is a common foot infection caused by fungi called dermatophytes. Found in many different places indoors and outdoors, dermatophytes are especially common in the warm, moist environments of

✔ Intense itching of the feet

✔ Cracked, blistered, or peeling areas of skin, especially between the toes

✔ Redness and scaling on the soles

pools, showers, locker rooms, and other sports facilities, where people walk with bare feet. Once dermatophytes contaminate the skin of a foot, the warm, moist environment of sweaty socks and shoes encourages them to grow.

Treating athlete's foot

If you think you have athlete's foot, first try a nonprescription antifungal ointment, cream, or powder, such as clotrimazole (Lotrimin AF, Mycelex, generic), terbinafine (Lamisil AT, Silka, generic), or miconazole (Lotrimin AF spray, Micatin, generic). It can take weeks for an infection to improve, and recurrences are common.

If your symptoms don't resolve after several weeks, consult a doctor, who may prescribe an oral antifungal medicine, such as itraconazole (Sporanox, generic) or terbinafine (Lamisil, generic).

Preventing further problems

You can help to prevent athlete's foot by keeping your feet clean and dry. More specifically, you can try the following:

- Wash your feet well every day and wear a clean pair of socks after your bath or shower.
- Take time to dry your feet thoroughly (including each toe and especially the webbed area between the toes) after you bathe, shower, or swim.
- If you use public pools or showers, wear flip-flops or sandals to prevent your bare feet from touching floors contaminated with fungi.
- Choose leather shoes rather than vinyl, since leather lets feet "breathe" so they are more likely to stay dry.
- Wear cotton socks to absorb sweat.
- If possible, don't wear the same pair of shoes two days in a row. Give shoes a 24-hour break between wearings to air out and dry out.
- Don't share shoes.

Contact dermatitis

As the name implies, contact dermatitis—a type of rash—occurs after a person's skin comes in contact with an offending substance. Contact dermatitis can be caused either by an allergic reaction or by simple irritation from things such as detergents or harsh soaps (see "Contact dermatitis triggers," page 9). All told, more than 3,700 contact allergens have been identified.

Poison ivy and poison oak are classic examples of allergens that can provoke allergic contact dermatitis. Brush against one of these plants and within a few days, you may develop itchy, red blisters. However, allergic contact dermatitis can also develop unexpectedly, even after you've been around a substance for some time with no problem. For instance, nail polish, nickel in jewelry, and certain medications—such as topical antibiotics and anesthetics—can suddenly cause a reaction.

▶ **Symptoms of contact dermatitis**

✔ Itchy, red skin

✔ Tiny bumps or blisters

✔ Crusted patches on the skin that, if infected, develop a wet (weeping) look

Treating contact dermatitis

The first step in treatment is to wash the area thoroughly with mild soap to remove any trace of the substance causing the reaction. Avoiding the trigger is the next step. If you can't determine the cause of the allergy or irritation, testing by an allergy specialist can help reveal the cause. Once you know the trigger and can avoid it, you might not need further treatment. Keep in mind that the route of exposure may not always be obvious; for example, the plant oils responsible for poison ivy may go first to the fur of your pet or the fabric of your gardening clothes and then transfer to the surface of your skin. Contact dermatitis usually clears up in about two to three weeks so long as you avoid further contact with the substance that caused it.

If further treatment is needed, wet dressings and soothing lotions can help ease itching and other

Contact dermatitis triggers

Thousands of substances can trigger contact dermatitis; the following are some of the most common.

Allergic contact dermatitis

- botanical-based cosmetics that contain substances such as tree oil, lavender, and peppermint
- corticosteroids
- cosmetics
- fragrances
- hair dyes
- lanolin
- nickel
- poison ivy, poison oak, and other plants
- rubber
- shaving lotion*
- sunscreen*
- topical anesthetics
- topical antibiotics (Neomycin, Bacitracin)

Irritant contact dermatitis

- acids and alkalis
- detergents
- environmental chemicals (such as insect spray)
- ethylene oxide
- oils and greases
- soaps
- solvents

*These can become a problem in the presence of sunlight.

symptoms. Other treatments for contact dermatitis include these:

Corticosteroid creams or ointments. Available over the counter in varying strengths, these products ease itching and swelling. But in most cases, only more potent, prescription-strength topical corticosteroids will really help.

Oral corticosteroids. For severe cases, your doctor may prescribe prednisone, which is usually tapered off gradually, over about 10 to 14 days, to prevent recurrence of the rash.

Antihistamines. Over-the-counter non-sedating antihistamines such as fexofenadine (Allegra, generic), loratadine (Claritin, generic), and cetirizine (Zyrtec) may help control itching.

Eczema (atopic dermatitis)

Eczema is a chronic inflammatory skin disease that affects 10% to 20% of children and 1% to 3% of adults. It often begins in infancy as an intensely itchy rash. Most people can't help scratching, which leads to fur-

ther irritation and the possibility of skin infection caused by injury to the skin. The injured skin develops chronic inflammation and its function as a barrier is impaired.

Close to 50% of people with eczema have a family history of allergic diseases.

Symptoms of eczema

- ✔ Patches of dry, intensely itchy skin that may become red, swollen, and painful
- ✔ Patches that ooze fluid and crust over
- ✔ Infection in areas damaged from scratching
- ✔ Thick, flaking, scaly, dry skin (chronic eczema)

Treating eczema

Treatment involves rehydrating the skin by soaking in warm (not hot) baths or showers and then promptly applying moisturizers with a low water content to lock in the moisture. Thick creams, such as Aquaphor, Aveeno Eczema Therapy, CeraVe, Eucerin, and Vanicream, do a good job, as does the new in-shower moisturizer made by Eucerin. Choose moisturizers without fragrances and preservatives.

Limit your use of soaps and shampoos to once or twice a week, since soap products make skin dryness even worse by removing natural oils from the skin. Cetaphil is one soap that is non-irritating and has no fragrance in it, and the company makes a product specifically for people with eczema.

Management also includes soothing the ferocious itch with regular use of long-acting non-sedating oral antihistamines such as over-the-counter cetirizine (Zyrtec) during the day, or sedating antihistamines like diphenhydramine (Benadryl) at bedtime, since they can also help with sleep.

If eczema is not controlled by moisturizers and antihistamines alone, then doctors will recommend a prescription or over-the-counter topical corticosteroid to reduce inflammation in the skin. The corticosteroid should not be applied at the same time of day as your moisturizer, because the moisturizer can block your skin's ability to absorb the anti-inflammatory cream.

Corticosteroid creams and ointments are effective, but a major drawback is that potent steroids cannot be used for more than a week or two on the face—where symptoms often appear—because they gradually thin the skin and cause small blood vessels to break. Long-term use can also cause loss of skin pigmentation. Avoid extended use in areas of the skin that are warm and moist, such as in skin folds, because of increased absorption. Several trials show that once eczema is controlled, people can take a proactive approach to prevent flare-ups by applying a topical corticosteroid twice a week to areas that have healed but are prone to eczema.

Severe cases of eczema are sometimes treated with medications that suppress the immune system's response, such as tacrolimus (Protopic) and pimecrolimus (Elidel). These medications can be used on the face and have proven effective in inhibiting inflammation, have fewer side effects than corticosteroids, and may lessen the need for them. They can be used alone or with corticosteroids.

Preventing further problems

To prevent or reduce eczema flare-ups:
- Avoid exposure to extreme temperatures, dry air, harsh soaps, perfumed products, and bubble baths.
- Use blankets and clothing made of cotton. Avoid more irritating fabrics, such as wool. Avoid stiff synthetics, such as polyester.
- After showering or bathing, pat dry (rather than rub). That way, you leave a little moisture on your skin. Then apply a moisturizing cream or lotion to trap moisture in the skin.
- Use a humidifier.

Drug-resistant skin infections

Skin infections are usually minor, causing small pimples or boils that go away without antibiotics. But a growing number of skin infections are severe or life-threatening and do not respond to most antibiotics.

Skin infection caused by a persistent bacterium called methicillin-resistant *Staphylococcus aureus*, or MRSA, is increasingly common in the general population, including previously healthy children and adults.

▶ Symptoms and complications of drug-resistant skin infections

- ✔ Large pimples or boils that are red, swollen, and painful or are filled with pus
- ✔ Painful red sores that look like spider bites
- ✔ Wound infections
- ✔ Blood infections
- ✔ Pneumonia
- ✔ Bone infections
- ✔ Heart valve infections

Treating drug-resistant skin infections

If you have symptoms of a skin infection, see a doctor right away. Treatment depends on the location and severity of the infection. For a local pimple, boil, or abscess, the doctor will probably surgically drain it and may prescribe antibiotics.

MRSA infections are resistant to antibiotics in the penicillin family, but sulfa drugs, clindamycin, and some tetracycline derivatives may be effective. If a doctor prescribes antibiotics, be sure to finish the entire prescription, even if the infection seems to be gone.

Preventing further problems

To guard against skin infections, practice good hygiene:
- Wash your hands frequently.
- Don't share personal items like towels or razors.
- Clean and cover any cuts or other skin wounds.

Dry skin

A lifetime of sun exposure damages skin, leaving it thinner and less likely to hold in moisture. Also, aging skin produces less of the natural oils that keep skin lubricated. Some medical conditions, such as hypothyroidism, diabetes, and kidney disease, increase the likelihood of developing dry skin.

▶ Symptoms of dry skin

- ✔ Scaly patches of skin, with or without redness
- ✔ Itching
- ✔ Overall dryness

Treating dry skin

The first line of defense against dry skin is a moisturizer that softens and smooths skin with water and lipids (fats). Some moisturizers attract water to the skin and seal it in, while others prevent skin from losing water by coating it with a thick, impermeable layer. Effective products include the following:

Petrolatum (petroleum jelly). This waxy, greasy substance—commonly known by its brand name, Vaseline—stops water loss without clogging pores. It can be used by itself, but is also a component of a number of moisturizers and ointments because it's inexpensive and effective. Because petroleum jelly doesn't contain water, it's best used while the skin is still damp after bathing to seal in moisture.

Oils. Moisturizing oils, such as mineral oil, have the same effect as petrolatum without being as greasy. Oils should also be used while the skin is still damp.

Emollient lotions and creams. These products contain both water and oils and are therefore less greasy and more cosmetically appealing than either petroleum jelly or oils. Most also contain an emulsifier to keep the product from separating.

Humectants, including sorbitol and glycerin, are used to bind water to the skin and help it absorb moisture. Look for moisturizers that contain at least one of the following ingredients: glycerin, urea, pyroglutamic acid, sorbitol, lactic acid, lactate salts, or alpha hydroxy acids.

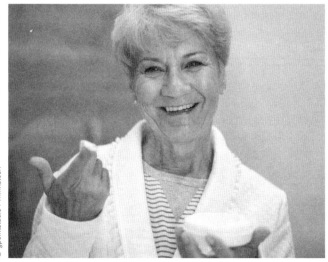

Aging skin produces less of the natural oils that keep skin lubricated. Your first line of defense against dry skin is a moisturizer.

Preventing further problems

The following changes to your lifestyle or environment can help alleviate dry skin:

- Add moisture to the air with a humidifier or a pan of water set atop the radiator.
- In the shower or bath, use water that's lukewarm instead of hot; hot water can further dry the skin by stripping it of natural oils.
- Choose nondrying soaps that contain no abrasives or irritants. Super-fatted soaps or cleansing bars are less drying than regular, liquid, or antibacterial soaps.
- Instead of rubbing, pat your skin dry after you bathe. Apply moisturizer immediately to retain the water your skin absorbed while bathing. Fast-drying moisturizers have recently become available that are applied by hand in the shower even before toweling off: Eucerin, Jergens, and Olay are popular brands. Spray-on moisturizers from St. Ives, Vaseline, and other companies are also available, but be careful to use them in a carpeted area, as they can make the floor slippery.
- Wear soft fabrics that won't scratch or irritate the skin.

Excess hair growth

An overgrowth of hair is called hypertrichosis. It is most common in women and often occurs around the time of menopause. Hypertrichosis is characterized by excessive growth in locations that already have fine, light-colored hair, such as the upper lip or along the jaw line. It differs from hirsutism, which causes women to develop male hair growth patterns, such as hair on the chest. While hypertrichosis is related to age and hormonal changes, hirsutism is caused by underlying endocrine disorders such as adrenal gland tumors or polycystic ovary syndrome. Regardless of the cause, excess hair growth can be embarrassing. A variety of solutions, including laser treatments, are available.

Treating excess hair growth

Temporary hair removal techniques include shaving, plucking, waxing, and using depilatories, which are chemical hair-removal products. In the past, the

✔ The appearance of thick dark hair in areas where light hair ordinarily grows

✔ An increase in dark hair on the body following menopause

only permanent means of removing excess hair was with electrolysis, which uses a shortwave electrical current to destroy the hair follicles. Newer techniques to reduce hair regrowth include the following light-based techniques:

Intense pulsed light (IPL). This uses a device that emits bursts of broadband light energy that are absorbed by the pigment in the hair. This turns the light into heat, which then damages the hair follicle. It works only on dark hair—not blond, red, gray, or white hair. IPL treatment should not be used on tanned or dark skin because it can cause temporary or permanent pigment changes in the skin.

Laser hair removal. This treatment uses lasers to destroy hair follicles by the same mechanism as described for IPL. Like IPL, it only works on dark hair. A single treatment destroys 10% to 20% of follicles in the area treated. Hair that does grow back is thinner and softer. After three treatments, about 60% of the hair may not grow back. The long-pulsed alexandrite and long-pulsed diode lasers work best for people with fair skin. Lasers with longer wavelengths, such as Nd:YAG lasers, are best for removing hair on people with tanned or darker skin. Brands include Apogee, GentleLase, GentleYAG, LightSheer Duet Diode, and Profile. (Also see "Home treatments and devices," page 48.)

For both laser hair removal and IPL, the cost depends on the size of the area being treated and the number of treatments required. For most people, three or more treatments are needed in order to achieve a noticeable reduction in hair regrowth. Rare complications include burning of the skin with blistering, herpes simplex outbreaks in people already carrying the virus, bacterial infections, and temporary skin lightening or darkening. To reduce your risk of complications, make sure the person performing your laser hair removal is licensed and experienced. Before

beginning treatment, avoid tanning and use a broad-spectrum sunscreen for up to six weeks.

Hair loss

It's normal to lose up to 100 hairs per day. But if you see lots of thinning or bald patches, you may have an inherited condition known as androgenic alopecia (also known as male-pattern or female-pattern baldness)—the most common cause of premature hair loss. Other factors that can cause hair loss include immune disorders, exposure to toxic chemicals, stress, burns, various skin disorders, and treatment with chemotherapy drugs. Many other medications, including some used to treat heart disease, depression, hormonal problems, and other conditions, can in rare cases cause hair loss.

Eyelash renewal

After people noticed that a prescription drug for glaucoma, bimatoprost (Lumigan), made eyelashes longer and thicker, makers of the drug sought (and received) FDA approval for a cosmetic prescription formulation of the drug. Marketed as Latisse, it costs about $140 for a month's supply. Side effects may include eye infections and allergic reactions.

In addition to eyelash renewal, the drug also has a couple "off-label" uses, meaning that doctors sometimes prescribe it for other conditions, even though it is only FDA-approved for eyelashes. Clinical trials have shown that bimatoprost is effective for regrowing hair on the scalp. It is also used off-label for thickening eyebrows.

Some nonprescription products for eyelash enhancement contain substances similar to bimatoprost, such as isopropyl cloprostenate and dechloro ethylcloprostenolamide. These have benefits and risks similar to Latisse. Other products containing a variety of different ingredients are said to promote eyelash growth or to "condition eyelashes." But these products are short on published scientific data to demonstrate their effectiveness or safety. Cosmetic products are generally unregulated by the FDA so long as they make no health claims or purport to alter the biological structures of the body. For example, to say a product "conditions eyelashes" is a way of promoting it without violating this federal regulation. But it does not mean that the product actually increases eyelash length or thickness as the prescription drug bimatoprost does.

Symptoms of hair loss

Hair loss may follow one of several patterns, depending on the cause:

- ✔ receding hairline and gradual loss of hair on top of the head
- ✔ even thinning of hair over much of the scalp
- ✔ scattered areas of hair loss

Treating hair loss

Options for treating hair loss include medicines and surgical procedures. You can also ask your doctor to take a close look at any medications or supplements you are taking that might contribute to hair loss and switch to an alternative drug, if possible.

Minoxidil (Rogaine, generic). Applied twice daily to the scalp, this nonprescription medicine is available in a 2%- or 5%-strength liquid or a 5%-strength foam. The 5% solution is more effective than the 2% liquid in both men and women. It stops hair from becoming thinner and stimulates hair growth on the top of the scalp.

Finasteride (Propecia). This prescription oral medicine lowers serum and tissue levels of one of the hormones associated with androgenic alopecia, but has only been proved effective in men and is not approved for women of childbearing age, as it may affect fetal development if a woman is pregnant. Some men choose to use finasteride and minoxidil at the same time, but it's not clear that this practice results in more or faster hair regrowth or retention.

Spironolactone (Aldactone, generic). This prescription drug is also used sometimes to treat hair loss in women. The drug isn't terribly effective and is not FDA-approved for this use, but it blocks the effects of androgens on the hair follicles and may work for some women who are producing an excess of these hormones.

Surgical treatments. One option is a hair transplant, which involves transplanting healthy hair follicles from other parts of the scalp to areas affected by baldness. This often requires two to three sessions, about four months apart. Other surgical procedures are scalp reduction (the removal of bald scalp patches, bringing hair-bearing areas of scalp closer together) and scalp flap surgery (moving hair-bearing segments of scalp to bald areas).

Psoriasis

Although classified as a skin disease, psoriasis actually starts inside the body, the result of an immune system abnormality. In about a third of cases, the immune problem is genetic. People with psoriasis often have family members with the disease. But other factors also play a role. Psoriasis has been linked to psychological stress, obesity, smoking, alcohol use, strep throat, viral infections, and certain medications, including beta blockers (used to treat high blood pressure) and lithium (prescribed for mood disorders).

Psoriasis can occur in different places on the body, with slightly different symptoms; the four variants of the disease are known as plaque, guttate, inverse, and pustular psoriasis (see "Symptoms of psoriasis," below).

Symptoms of psoriasis

- ✔ Itchy, dry, cracked skin that may bleed
- ✔ Sharply defined, salmon-pink plaques covered with silver scales, most often on the elbows, knees, or scalp or near the buttocks, and sometimes on the trunk, arms, and legs (plaque psoriasis)
- ✔ Numerous small red scaly spots scattered on the arms and legs (guttate psoriasis)
- ✔ Smooth patches of red, inflamed skin in the creases of the underarms, groin, buttocks, or genital area or under the breasts (inverse psoriasis)
- ✔ Skin patches stuffed with pimples or pustules (pustular psoriasis)
- ✔ Thickened, pitted, or ridged nails

Treating psoriasis

Very mild cases may improve with moisturizers and some sunlight. But most people need other treatments, such as the following:

Ointments, gels, or lotions. The most common are corticosteroids, which come in varying strengths. They quickly lessen inflammation and control itching, but long-term use of strong steroids can thin and damage skin. Prescription therapies include calcipotriene (Dovonex, generic), a vitamin D derivative; tazarotene (Tazorac), a vitamin A relative; and a combination of a corticosteroid and calcipotriene (Taclonex, generic).

Phototherapy. This treatment, for moderate to severe psoriasis, uses carefully controlled exposure to ultraviolet (UV) light, sometimes together with a light-sensitizing medication called psoralen that makes the skin more responsive to UV light. Laser light, which allows for more focused, higher levels of UV light, may also be used. UV light helps slow the growth of skin cells.

Systemic therapy. Serious cases may require systemic therapies (that is, treatments that affect the entire body), including an oral vitamin A–like drug called acitretin (Soriatane); an injectable medication used to treat cancer and rheumatoid arthritis called methotrexate (Rheumatrex, Trexall); and oral cyclosporine (Gengraf, Neoral, others), which suppresses the immune system. These drugs can be toxic and can't be used for extended periods of time. Apremilast (Otezla), a newer oral treatment that targets molecules inside immune cells and thus regulates inflammation, helps both psoriatic arthritis and psoriasis.

Biologic drugs, which alter the immune response, can also help to control severe psoriasis. The injectable drugs etanercept (Enbrel), adalimumab (Humira), ustekinumab (Stelara), and the infusible drug infliximab (Remicade) have been used for several years. Now, other biologics that are even more effective are being introduced, such as ixekizumab (Taltz), which you inject every two weeks for 12 weeks and then every four weeks thereafter. In three clinical trials, participants who gave themselves ixekizumab injections were much more likely to achieve clear or almost-clear skin than those on a placebo. Secukinumab (Cosentyx) has also been approved by the FDA, and another new drug, brodalumab, passed an FDA advisory committee in July 2016.

The advantages of biologics are that you can stay on them for a longer time (the ixekizumab trials lasted five years) and there is no need to have routine blood tests as you do with the older, more toxic drugs. The pharmaceutical companies that make them have also established free nursing services over the telephone and in person to answer questions and instruct you in giving yourself the injections.

Rosacea

Rosacea is characterized by flare-ups of reddened and sometimes bumpy facial skin, mainly in the middle of the face but sometimes over the entire face. In rare cases, the eyes or scalp may also be affected. It's not clear what causes the condition, but genes and environmental exposures seem to play a role. Some experts think that exposure to certain mites or bacteria may trigger it by causing inflammation. Rosacea runs in families.

▶ Symptoms of rosacea
✔ Flushing of the face and neck
✔ Pimples
✔ Enlarged blood vessels (called telangiectasia)
✔ Redness and swelling of the nose
✔ Irritation of the eyes

Treating rosacea
Rosacea has no cure, but you can control symptoms by avoiding anything that increases blood flow to the face, including hot drinks, alcohol, spicy foods, hot baths or showers, and rubbing your face. Avoid lotions and cosmetics that contain alcohol and fragrances. Vanicream is a line of products that is useful for people with rosacea.

Several treatments can help control redness and pimples and prevent the most severe symptoms—enlarged blood vessels and swelling and thickening of the skin of the nose or chin. Depending on your symptoms, your doctor may prescribe one of the following:

Creams and gels. The topical antibiotic metronidazole (MetroCream, MetroGel, generic) is a common first-line treatment. Another option is azelaic acid (Azelex, Finacea) for the inflammatory pimples of mild to moderate rosacea. The newest cream and perhaps the most effective is ivermectin (Soolantra), which has both anti-inflammatory and antiparasitic properties.

A drug called brimonidine (Mirvaso) can be used to temporarily improve the appearance of facial redness by constricting blood vessels. In some people, though, the skin may actually become too pale, and some patients get post-treatment flares of rosacea, so use of this medication has become less frequent. However, other topical medications that achieve the same effect without side effects are in development.

Low-dose oral antibiotics. Doxycycline (available under various brand names and as a generic), often used in low-dose, delayed-absorption formulations, and other antibiotics can help quell rosacea's inflammation. Some people start with both oral and topical antibiotics and then move to using just topical treatments.

Laser treatments. This therapy damages or destroys the blood vessels that cause red lines and blotches. Effective treatments include the pulsed dye laser (yellow light), pulsed green-light laser, and intense pulsed light. Several treatments are usually required, spaced six to 12 weeks apart.

Shingles (herpes zoster)

If you, like most adults, had chickenpox as child, the varicella-zoster virus responsible for the infection probably remains in your body, lying dormant in one of your spinal nerves. Shingles occurs when the virus becomes active again later in life and causes a painful rash. Not everyone who has had chickenpox develops shingles, but up to one in five people in the United States will get shingles at some point. It's most common in people older than 50 and those with weakened immune systems (for example, in people undergoing cancer treatment).

Shingles starts with a burning sensation, a mild itching or tingling, or a shooting pain in a large patch of skin—usually on one side of the torso or face, or on a portion of an arm or leg. The skin may be extremely sensitive, so that you may not be able to stand even the touch of clothing on the area.

After about five days, the skin becomes red and mildly swollen, and a rash appears. Blisters may cluster in patches or form a continuous line that roughly follows the path of the infected nerve. The blisters may be painful or itchy, and some may be as large as the palm of your hand. Blisters continue to appear over two to seven days and eventually break, form crusts, and then heal.

About 10% of people who get shingles go on to develop postherpetic neuralgia, which causes long-term pain in the area where the blisters occurred, even after the rash has healed completely. Severe pain is most common in older people and often is accompanied by extreme sensitivity to heat and cold in the affected area of skin.

▶ Symptoms of shingles

- ✔ Tingling, itching sensation on skin, usually located only on one side of the torso or face or on a portion of an arm or leg
- ✔ Sharp burning pain on skin
- ✔ Clusters of small fluid-filled sacs
- ✔ Extreme sensitivity to touch, so much that you can't stand clothing touching or rubbing the area
- ✔ In some people, chills, fever, nausea, or diarrhea preceding other symptoms

Treating shingles

If you suspect that you have shingles, see a doctor immediately for treatment to shorten the course of the condition, minimize pain, and reduce the risk for nerve damage. Keeping the skin clean is important to avoid secondary bacterial infection. Applying cool compresses also may help ease the discomfort.

Treatments include these:

Analgesics. Pain-relieving drugs such as ibuprofen (Advil, generic) or acetaminophen (Tylenol, generic) may help reduce pain and discomfort.

Oral antiviral drugs. These drugs—acyclovir (Zovirax, generic), famciclovir (Famvir, generic), and valacyclovir (Valtrex, generic)—are most helpful when given within 72 hours of when the rash first appears. They may help lower the risk of postherpetic neuralgia.

Preventing shingles

People ages 50 and older can get a vaccine called Zostavax, which cuts the risk of shingles by half and lowers the risk of postherpetic neuralgia if you do get shingles. The vaccine contains the same ingredients as the chickenpox vaccine for children, but the dose is 14 times stronger. It is not effective for people who already have shingles or postherpetic neuralgia—but once your infection has cleared, you can receive the vaccine in the hopes of preventing future episodes. It's too soon to know if the standard chickenpox vaccine for children (which became available in 1995) will prevent shingles later in life.

The optimal age for vaccination is unknown, and there are no data to show how long protection lasts if you get the vaccine in your 50s; it's also not known if you can be safely reinoculated. A study of the vaccine, called the Shingles Prevention Study, tested only people who were over age 60 and found its effectiveness decreased during the five years after vaccination. Because of this, the CDC recommends vaccination for people 60 and older, under the assumption that the greatest risk for shingles occurs in that decade of life.

A newer two-dose vaccine called Shingrix is in late-stage clinical trials and may be even more effective than Zostavax, reducing the risk of shingles by as much as 97% in people 50 and older. Zostavax reduces the risk by just 50% in adults ages 50 to 69, and it loses its effectiveness in people over age 70—meaning the older you are when you get the currently available vaccine, the less likely it is to protect you from shingles.

Toenail fungus

Fungi that thrive in the dark, moist, and stuffy environment inside shoes are responsible for this unsightly condition. The fungi feed on keratin, the protein that makes up the hard surface of the toenails. Anyone can get toenail fungus, but it's more common in older people, as well as those who have chronic illnesses such as diabetes or circulatory problems that decrease blood flow to the toes. The fungus may spread on the floors of showers and locker rooms, just like the fungus that causes athlete's foot (see page 7). Wearing tight-fitting shoes and heavy layers of nail polish (which doesn't let the nail breathe) also increase the risk of this infection. The big toe and smallest toe are the most likely to

become infected, perhaps because they're exposed to friction from the sides of shoes.

▶ Symptoms of toenail fungus

Toenails may become

- ✔ yellow or brown-colored
- ✔ white, soft, and powdery
- ✔ thickened or overgrown
- ✔ brittle, crumbly, or ragged

Treating toenail fungus

Many treatments for toenail fungus exist, but their effectiveness and cost vary widely. And unfortunately, the infection often recurs.

Antifungal creams or solutions. Over-the-counter products that claim to treat toenail fungus rarely work, except perhaps for very mild cases that only affect a single toe.

Vicks VapoRub. This pungent-smelling product is one of many home remedies suggested for treating toenail fungus. Others include vinegar, Listerine, and tea tree oil. Two small studies suggest Vicks actually does help—one reported that 38% of people had no more fungus after using the medicated rub on the affected toenails for five to 16 months.

Topical nail solutions. Ciclopirox (Penlac), efinaconazole (Jublia), and tavaborole (Kerydin) are prescription antifungal medications that are applied daily with a brush or dropper. Complete treatment takes almost a year, and many people have trouble faithfully applying the medication for that long. During treatment, you will also need to trim your toenails weekly. Only about one in 15 people sees favorable results with ciclopirox; the other two drugs are much more effective. Topical nail solutions can be costly, though, and are not typically covered by insurance since toenail fungus is considered to be a cosmetic issue.

Oral antifungal medications. Prescription antifungal drugs such as terbinafine (Lamisil, generic) and itraconazole (Sporanox, generic) taken daily for several months cure most cases (60% to 70%). But even after your toenails grow out, they may never become clear or normal-looking. These medications also have uncommon—but serious—side effects, including liver damage, so your doctor will monitor you while you're using them.

Laser or photodynamic therapy. Limited data suggest a benefit from a series of laser treatments or photodynamic therapy (see page 49) of infected toenails. But these therapies, performed by dermatologists or podiatrists, are costly and are not reliably effective.

Surgery. For very severe cases that don't respond to other treatment, doctors sometimes surgically remove the entire nail or nails.

Preventing further problems

Follow these steps to help prevent toenail fungus:

- Wear comfortable shoes and hosiery that allow your feet some breathing space.
- Wear shoes, sandals, or flip-flops in community showers or locker rooms.
- Wash your feet every day. Dry them thoroughly, and use an antifungal or antibiotic foot powder.
- Wear clean socks or stockings every day.
- Keep your toenails trimmed.
- Disinfect pedicure tools before you use them.

Warts

Warts are small skin growths caused by an infection of the top layer of the skin with human papillomavirus (HPV). Common skin warts appear mainly on the hands and arms, while plantar warts occur on the feet (see the lists of symptoms, below). Genital warts appear on and near the genitals (see "Genital warts," below). The virus can be transmitted from one person to another either by direct contact or indirectly when both people come in contact with the same surface, such as a floor or desk. Warts can appear at any age but are more common in older children and are uncommon in the elderly.

Most warts go away after a year or two and are little more than an inconvenience. But some last for years or come back after going away. Warts that persist or grow despite treatment should be examined by your doctor, since some skin cancers can masquerade as warts.

▶ Symptoms of common skin warts

- ✔ Raised round or oval growths the size of a pencil eraser or smaller
- ✔ Often on the fingers, hands, knees, and elbows
- ✔ Light gray, flesh-colored, yellow, brown, or gray-black

▶ Symptoms of plantar warts

- ✔ Flattened growths on the soles of the feet
- ✔ Sometimes painful, especially when on a weight-bearing part of the foot

Genital warts

Genital warts can appear on or near the genitals and in the anus in both men and women, as well as inside the vagina and on the cervix in women. They look like small, flesh-colored bumps that may have a cauliflower-like appearance, though some are too small to see. Symptoms can include itching or discomfort in the genital areas and bleeding with intercourse, although some infected people have no symptoms.

Treatments include cryotherapy (see page 18) and topical prescription creams such as imiquimod (Aldara, Zyclara, generic), and podofilox (Condylox, generic), which people can apply themselves. The newest topical medication is an ointment made from an extract of green tea leaves; it is called sinecatechins (Veregen) and is available only by prescription. Stronger treatments such as trichloroacetic acid must be applied by a doctor. Do not use over-the counter treatments designed for other types of warts, as these are not intended to be used in the sensitive genital area. Larger or stubborn warts may require surgery or laser treatments.

Avoiding all sexual contact is the only sure way to prevent genital warts, but using condoms may lower the risk. Vaccines (Cervarix, Gardasil, Gardasil 9) protect against the strains of HPV that are known to cause cervical cancer. Gardasil and Gardasil 9 also protect against the HPV strains that are responsible for most genital warts. The vaccines are given as a series of three shots and are recommended for boys and girls starting at age 11 or 12 and certain other groups of people up to age 26; see the CDC's website at www.cdc.gov/hpv/prevention.html for more information.

Treating warts

Many warts respond to at-home treatments. However, if you have diabetes or neuropathy (nerve damage), check with a doctor before trying any of these treatments yourself.

Salicylic acid. Available over the counter as a liquid or in a patch (Clear Away, Compound W, others), this acid helps to remove warts. For best results, soak the wart in water for 10 to 20 minutes to soften the skin, then dry before applying the medicine. Between treatments, use a nail file or pumice stone to slough off dead skin from the wart's surface. You may need to apply the medication every day for weeks or months to clear a wart.

Duct tape. This sticky, silver tape has proved effective in removing warts, although study findings have been mixed. You cover the wart with tape and leave it in place for six days, remove the tape, soak the area for 10 to 20 minutes, then slough off the skin with a pumice stone. Leave the skin uncovered overnight, then reapply tape for another six days. Most people who find this treatment helpful see results within about two weeks, but complete disappearance of the wart can take up to a month.

If you consult a doctor, he or she may recommend one of these treatments:

Cryotherapy. The most common wart treatment, cryotherapy is done in a doctor's office and uses liquid nitrogen to freeze off the wart. The treatment stings, and more than one application is often needed.

Curettage. A doctor removes the wart with a curved blade after numbing the skin.

Creams and liquids. Different prescription medications (applied in a doctor's office or at home) can treat skin warts. Some work by stimulating the immune system to eliminate HPV. Pain and irritation can occur, and these medications aren't terribly effective.

Injected yeast. A doctor can inject *Candida albicans*, commonly known as yeast, into a wart to stimulate a local immune response and clear the wart. Side effects are mild. ❦

Skin cancer

Those carefree days you spent sunning and swimming as a child may have caused more damage than the lines and wrinkles of photoaging. They may have also set the stage for skin cancer.

Skin cancer is the most common cancer in the United States, causing about 13,650 deaths annually. Most of these deaths (about 10,130) are from melanoma, the most severe form of skin cancer, which has become far more common as people have spent more leisure time outdoors. The other two types of skin cancer are squamous cell carcinoma and basal cell carcinoma (see Figure 3). The good news is that with early detection and treatment, more than 90% of cases can be cured, although the results can be disfiguring. Doctors can also treat a precancerous condition called actinic keratosis.

Figure 3: Three kinds of skin cancer

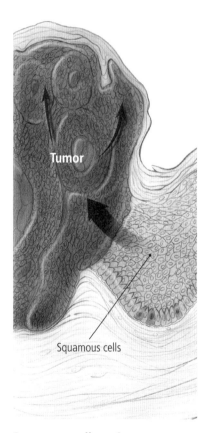 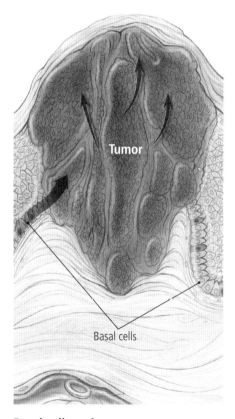 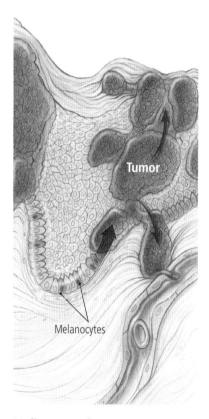

Squamous cell carcinoma

This type of cancer begins in the middle portion of the epidermis and affects only the surrounding area, but it eventually forms a raised patch with a rough surface.

Basal cell carcinoma

The cells of this type of cancer resemble the cells in the lowest layer of the epidermis, the basal layer. The malignant cells invade surrounding tissues, forming a painless bump that later becomes an open ulcer with a hard edge.

Malignant melanoma

The deadliest form of skin cancer occurs when melanocytes—pigment-making cells in the basal layer or in surface moles—begin reproducing uncontrollably. Left untreated, the cancer can spread to distant parts of the body.

On the prevention side, regular use of sunscreen and sun avoidance significantly reduce the risk of skin cancer, and daily sunscreen use alone can cut the risk of melanoma in half.

Actinic keratosis

Actinic keratosis (AK) is a precancerous skin condition that appears as scaly pink or red-brown raised, rough patches on sun-exposed skin. Fair-skinned people are more likely than darker-complexioned individuals to develop AK. The condition can cause discomfort and itching, but its biggest danger is as a precursor to squamous cell carcinoma. Most treatments can remove AK spots without scarring.

▶ Symptoms of actinic keratosis

✔ Rough, scaly red or brown patch on skin

✔ Most likely to appear on face, back of hands, or other areas commonly exposed to sun

Treating actinic keratosis

Doctors can use several different methods to remove areas of actinic keratosis.

Cryotherapy. The standard treatment for AK is to freeze the area with liquid nitrogen. Inflammation, swelling, and occasionally blistering may occur. A small scab forms, and healthy new skin emerges as it heals. Cryotherapy can be used to treat a specific lesion or multiple lesions.

Creams and gels. The prescription gel ingenol mebutate (Picato) can be applied for three consecutive days on the scalp and face to remove AK spots. Alternatively, a prescription cream containing the chemotherapy drug fluorouracil, also called 5-FU (Carac, Efudex, Fluoroplex), can be used once or twice a day for several weeks or on two consecutive days a week for several months. Another topically applied drug, called imiquimod (Aldara, Zyclara, generic), is also very effective in treating AK spots. Imiquimod stimulates the immune system to release cytokines, chemicals that fight cancer cells and viruses. Imiquimod causes AK patches to become inflamed, crust over, and heal. All of these products cause an inflammatory reaction in the skin, resulting in temporary redness and discomfort. In addition, products containing fluorouracil cause sun sensitivity. In contrast, a topical gel called diclofenac (Solaraze, generic) does not cause redness, but requires months of treatment.

Deeper treatments. Widespread facial patches may warrant deeper treatments such as laser resurfacing (see page 44) with a carbon dioxide, erbium:YAG, or fractional 1927 nm laser or a strong chemical peel containing trichloroacetic acid, which dissolves the outer layers of the skin with a chemical solution. Laser resurfacing and chemical peels can involve local or general anesthesia. Depending on how deeply the skin is penetrated, they may cause considerable swelling. Still another effective treatment is curettage with electrodesiccation, which entails scraping away damaged tissue and using an electric probe to kill any remaining cancerous cells.

Photodynamic therapy. This treatment uses light to activate a therapeutic agent. In this case, the agent is Levulan, a topical solution of aminolevulinic acid—an acid that occurs naturally in the body to process heme, a component of red blood cells. First, Levulan is applied to AK spots, where it changes into a light-sensitive molecule. Several hours to a day later, light or laser treatment activates the drug and destroys the AK cells. In a few days, the spots crust over and heal. Photodynamic therapy is used in cases where someone has many AK spots and whole areas of the face and scalp need to be treated.

Basal cell and squamous cell carcinomas

Both these types of skin cancer have been on the rise for many years. This is probably because of increased detection, more sun exposure, and an aging population. More than three million men and women are diagnosed with nonmelanoma skin cancer in the United States each year. But only about 2,000 people die from these cancers annually, and most of these deaths are among people whose immune systems are compromised by age or disease.

The most benign form of skin cancer—and the least likely to spread to other parts of the body—is basal cell carcinoma. It's also the most common form, accounting for about 80% of cases. Basal cell carcinoma originates in basal cells located deep in the epidermis. The most common cause of this cancer is cumulative damage from sun exposure. A basal cell carcinoma may first appear as a pearly pimple or bump, a white- or yellow-colored scar, or a scaly red patch. Some basal cell cancers appear as an ulcer that won't heal. Basal cell cancer is very slow-growing and will not develop into melanoma, the most deadly form of skin cancer.

About 20% of skin cancers are squamous cell carcinomas. This form of cancer arises from flat, scale-like cells in the epidermis. Although squamous cell cancer usually isn't fatal, it can be life-threatening if it spreads to lymph nodes or internal organs. But even then, the cure rate is around 50%. Four times more men than women develop squamous cell carcinoma. It usually starts as a small, scaly bump and grows slowly until it resembles an ulcer or wart. Squamous cell cancers frequently occur on the face, lips, ears, or backs of the hands, and they too result from cumulative sun damage. Early detection is key to preventing the spread of squamous cell cancer. Like basal cell cancer, it will not develop into melanoma.

▶ Symptoms of basal cell carcinoma
- ✔ Small, smooth white or pink bump
- ✔ May become an ulcer or open sore
- ✔ Less commonly, a small, flat, red spot or recurring scar

▶ Symptoms of squamous cell carcinoma
- ✔ Raised crusty bump
- ✔ Size ranges from that of a pea to a walnut
- ✔ Less often, a flat or slightly elevated area of skin

Treating basal cell and squamous cell cancers

Options for treating basal and squamous cell cancers are similar. Which treatment is best for you depends on factors such as the size and location of the cancer, whether it has returned after earlier treatment, and your age and general health. If surgery is required, the tumor is carefully removed along with the tissue around it, called the margin, to ensure that all cancer cells have been eradicated. If they haven't, another procedure will be required. Most experienced dermatologists are quite skilled at estimating appropriate margins. The surgical scar can take several months to heal, especially if a tumor was removed from the face.

The following surgical and medical options are among the wide range of treatments available.

Excision. The cancerous tissue is cut away along with a small (3- to 10-millimeter) margin of healthy tissue. Then the skin is stitched closed with sutures. If a large area of skin is removed, skin from elsewhere in the body can be used to cover the area (a skin graft).

Curettage and electrodesiccation. The cancerous tissue is scraped away, and an electrode is used to kill any remaining microscopic cancerous cells.

Cryosurgery. Freezing the cancerous tissues with liquid nitrogen kills them. This treatment usually is reserved for precancers or very small tumors.

Radiation. The cancerous tissue is destroyed with a series of high-energy rays aimed from outside the body.

Mohs micrographic surgery. The tumor is shaved away in thin layers, one layer at a time, and each layer is checked immediately under a microscope. This allows the surgeon to preserve as much healthy skin as possible while making sure that all of the cancer is removed. This is the most common treatment for skin cancers on delicate or small areas such as the face and fingers.

Other treatments. These include anticancer drugs such as fluorouracil or imiquimod applied directly to the skin.

Melanoma

Melanoma is a form of cancer that originates in the melanocytes, cells deep in the epidermis, or in surface moles that produce pigment. Although melanoma accounts for only about 1% of cases of skin cancer, it's responsible for the vast majority of all skin cancer deaths. An estimated 76,380 new cases of melanoma will be diagnosed in the United States in 2016. Without early detection and treatment, it can spread (metastasize) to the lymph nodes and internal organs. The lungs and liver are common targets when melanoma spreads.

Melanoma has been on the increase for at least three decades, but it is much more common in whites than in people with darker skin. Over all, the lifetime risk of getting melanoma is about 2.5% for whites (one in 40) but only 0.1% for blacks and 0.5% for Hispanics. It is slightly more common in men than in women.

Your risk of developing melanoma is higher if you have

- red or blond hair
- green or blue eyes
- fair skin
- a history of being in the sun a lot, especially as a child

▶ Symptoms of melanoma

If a spot on your skin meets any of the criteria below, be sure to see a dermatologist right away.

 Asymmetry. Most moles have a round, symmetrical shape, but melanoma is asymmetrical, meaning one side may be different in shape than the other.

 Border irregularity. Normal moles are round and typically have a clear border. In melanoma, the borders are shabby, uneven, or indistinct, sometimes blending into the surrounding skin. A mole resembling the shape of cauliflower, for instance, should be checked out.

 Color. Melanomas are usually very dark, but often are a mix of hues rather than one color.

 Diameter. Most common moles are small, less than 6 millimeters, which is about a quarter of an inch. Melanoma grows, so talk to your doctor if the spot is larger than that.

Evolving. Look for any change in size, shape, color, or elevation, or any new symptoms such as bleeding, itching, or crusting.

- a mother, father, sister, or brother with melanoma; if one of these relatives has melanoma, you are eight times more likely to develop it.

Features of freckles or moles that raise your risk of melanoma include

- a new mole appearing after age 30
- a new mole at any age if it is in an area rarely exposed to the sun
- a change in an existing mole
- one or more atypical moles—moles that look like a fried egg or moles that are darker than others or have irregular borders or an irregular shape
- 20 or more moles larger than 2 millimeters across
- five or more moles larger than 5 millimeters across
- freckles caused by being in the sun.

Melanoma has several distinguishing characteristics that experts call the ABCDEs (see "Symptoms of melanoma," at left). A mole or growth is considered suspicious if it is asymmetrical, meaning that one half of the growth looks different from the other; if its borders are irregular, ragged, or blurry; if its color is unusual; if its diameter exceeds 6 millimeters, about that of a pencil eraser; or if it has evolved, enlarged, or changed in any way. A dermatologist should examine a mole or growth with any of those characteristics.

Dermatologists commonly use dermoscopy to diagnose skin cancer. A dermatoscope is a small handheld microscope that is placed close to or lightly against the skin to reveal pigment patterns in the lesion. Dermoscopy allows doctors to see extra details that are not visible to the naked eye, helping to differentiate suspicious moles from other pigmented lesions.

Treating melanoma

If a growth or mole looks like a melanoma, the doctor will take a biopsy to confirm the diagnosis. This entails removing either a sample of tissue or else the entire growth and some surrounding skin, and examining the tissue under a microscope to determine whether it's cancer. Depending on how deep a melanoma is, additional tissue may have to be removed. In some cases, lymph nodes may be removed, too. A procedure called a sentinel node biopsy can show whether the lymph node nearest the tumor contains any cancer cells. If it does, surgery to remove additional nodes right away can improve survival.

In addition to surgery, treatments for melanoma include immunotherapy (which strengthens the immune system against the cancer), chemotherapy, and radiation therapy. What's more, certain drugs can be used in combination with other treatments to stop the progression of the cancer and extend survival by months or even years. For example, immune checkpoint inhibitors such as pembrolizumab (Keytruda), nivolumab (Opdivo), and ipilimumab (Yervoy) are used for people with advanced disease. These drugs remove proteins that would otherwise hinder the immune system from clearing melanoma cells. Now researchers are studying whether these drugs can be given before or after melanoma surgery to prevent the cancer from recurring.

Newer, so-called targeted treatments home in on specific genetic changes seen in people with certain forms of melanoma. For example, about half of melanomas have genetic changes (mutations) in a gene called BRAF, which signals melanoma cells to grow and divide quickly. Drugs that inhibit BRAF, such as vemurafenib (Zelboraf) and dabrafenib (Tafinlar), and those that target related proteins called MEK proteins, such as trametinib (Mekinist) and cobimetinib (Cotellic), are now available to shrink melanomas.

These targeted treatments may have fewer side effects than chemotherapy drugs and work when chemotherapy doesn't. On the downside, they may work for only a short period of time and then stop being effective, although they may work longer if they're used in combination. Another genetic defect, in a gene called C-KIT, is associated with a small number of melanomas. The drug imatinib (Gleevec), dasatinib (Sprycel), and nilotinib (Tasigna) are being tested against C-KIT changes in clinical trials, while axitinib (Inlyta), pazopanib (Votrient), and everolimus (Afinitor) are being studied for their ability to target other defective genes and proteins.

Another exciting advance is in the area of vaccines. Several melanoma vaccines—designed both to prevent melanoma and to treat existing cases—are now being tested in clinical trials.

About 84% of people diagnosed with melanoma of the skin have stage 1 or localized melanoma, meaning the disease has not spread beyond its original site. For them, the five-year survival rate is about 95%. But if the cancer spreads to the lymph nodes (stage 3), five-year survival drops to between 40% and 78%. As with most other forms of cancer, if the tumor has spread to distant organs (stage 4), overall survival is still lower—about 15% to 20%. In short, as with most diseases, the earlier melanoma is detected and treated, the better the outcome. ▼

Protecting your skin

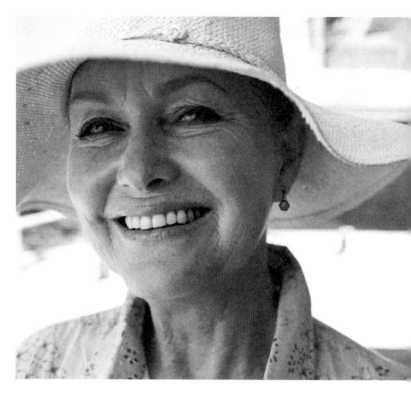

The single most important thing you can do to protect your skin is to reduce sun exposure. That means using sunscreen, wearing protective clothing, and limiting your time outdoors when the sun is strongest. Beyond that, there are steps you can take to manage the problems of aging skin, ranging from dryness to wrinkles. To keep your skin looking its best, take care to treat it gently, keep it hydrated, and report any changes you notice to your doctor immediately.

While the sun's ultraviolet (UV) rays are by far the biggest factor leading to skin damage, several other factors can also contribute. Here's a rundown of the key hazards, starting with sunlight, and what to do about them.

Sun damage

Sun damage is responsible for photoaging, the leading cause of skin damage as you age. For enthusiasts of the great outdoors, sun protection is not an easy task. But careful selection and application of a sunscreen can go a long way toward preventing further skin damage (see "How to use sunscreen," page 25). It's also important to wear protective hats and other clothing when outdoors in the sun. Choose a hat with a wide brim that extends two to three inches to shade your neck, nose, and ears (a baseball cap doesn't cut it). Also wear clothes with a tight weave, long sleeves, and long legs. Companies such as Coolibar and Sun Precautions/Solumbra make special sun-protective clothing.

But even the most scrupulous use of sunscreens and protective clothing is not as effective as minimizing exposure to dangerous UV light in the first place. The sun's rays are most intense between 10 a.m. and 2 p.m., so if you're going to be spending time outside, try to do so in the early morning or late afternoon. Stay in the shade when possible, and be aware of reflected light from water, sand, and snow (in winter).

Don't forget to look after the younger generation as well by protecting your children or grandchildren from sun exposure. Most sun damage that leads to skin cancer occurs early in life.

© I Thinkstock

Medications

If you're taking certain medications, sun exposure can cause additional damage to your skin. Such drugs, called photosensitizers, increase your sensitivity to UV radiation. Reactions include overly reddened skin, hives, swelling, and itchy, scaly skin. Cataracts and damage to blood vessels or the immune system also may occur.

Some of these drugs, such as heart medications, are more commonly taken by people as they get older. It's important to check with your doctor to determine whether any of the drugs you're taking could cause photosensitivity. (For a list of the most common offenders, see "Some medications that can cause photosensitivity," page 26.)

Infrared radiation

A less common cause of skin damage is exposure to infrared radiation (heat). It's not a major cause of skin damage, but researchers believe that it may add to the effects of UV rays. Some exposures may occur on the job—think of the short-order cook who stands over a hot stove or in front of infrared heat lamps all day. Infrared heat lamps also are used to heal some muscle injuries or to relieve pain and stiffness from osteoarthritis.

Cigarettes

Cigarette smoking has long been recognized as a cause of wrinkles. Tobacco smoke exposure decreases blood flow in the smaller vessels,

How to use sunscreen

Choosing the right sun protection and applying it properly are the most important steps you can take to protect your skin from the sun's harmful rays. It sounds simple, but these steps are often misunderstood. Here are the basics:

- Use a broad-spectrum, water-resistant sunscreen with an SPF of 30 to 50.
- Both chemical sunscreens (which contain compounds such as oxybenzone, avobenzone, ecamsule, padimate O, PABA, octyl methoxycinnamate, and octyl salicylate among others that absorb the sun's rays) and mineral sunscreens (which contain zinc oxide or titanium dioxide to physically block ultraviolet radiation) are acceptable.
- About two tablespoons (six teaspoons) is enough sunscreen for the average adult body, with about one teaspoon allotted for just your face.
- Apply sunscreen about 15 minutes before going out in the sun and reapply it every couple of hours.

In 2013, new labels began appearing on sunscreen bottles, per orders from the FDA. Some of the changes affect the terms permitted on labels. The term "sunblock" is no longer allowed; nor are the descriptions "sweat proof" and "waterproof." Instead, a sunscreen can be called "water resistant," but only for either 40 or 80 minutes—and only if it passes an FDA test.

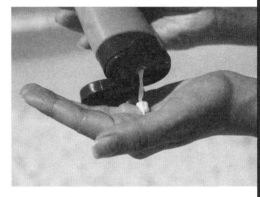

But the more important terms focus on what sunscreen can prevent. For a label to claim the sunscreen can prevent sunburn, the product must pass the sun protection factor (SPF) test. This test shows how long a sunscreen protects you from ultraviolet B (UVB) rays that cause sunburn. SPF levels range from 2 to more than 70. The higher the number, the longer the protection lasts. Say, for example, your skin turns red after 10 minutes in the sun. Sunscreen with an SPF of 15 would prevent your skin from turning red for 150 minutes under the same conditions.

You might think that an SPF of 30 would work twice as well as an SPF of 15. But that's not necessarily the case. While SPF 15 filters out approximately 93% of all incoming UVB rays, SPF 30 filters out 97%, and SPF 50 boosts that to 98%.

The American Academy of Dermatology (AAD) recommends using a broad-spectrum, water-resistant sunscreen with an SPF of at least 30. According to both the AAD and the FDA, you don't need a sunscreen with an SPF higher than 50, because there's no evidence that products with higher SPFs offer any additional protection.

For a product to claim it can prevent skin cancer, it must pass the broad-spectrum test. This shows whether a sunscreen can protect your skin from ultraviolet A (UVA) radiation, which contributes to skin cancer and early skin aging, as well as UVB rays.

© boophotography | Thinkstock

Some medications that can cause photosensitivity

- **Acne medications:** acitretin (Soriatane), isotretinoin (Accutane)

- **Antibiotics:** ciprofloxacin (Cipro, Proquin), doxycycline (Oracea, Vibramycin), sulfamethoxazole (Gantanol), sufamethoxazole and trimethoprim (Bactrim, Septra), tetracycline (Achromycin)

- **Antihistamines:** diphenhydramine (Benadryl)

- **Chemotherapy drugs:** 5-fluorouracil (Carac, Efudex, Fluoroplex), dacarbazine (DTIC-Dome)

- **Diabetes medications:** chlorpropamide (Diabinese), glyburide (DiaBeta, Glynase, Micronase)

- **Diuretics:** furosemide (Lasix), hydrochlorothiazide (Microzide)

- **Heart medications:** amiodarone (Cordarone), diltiazem (Cardizem, Dilacor, Tiazac), nifedipine (Procardia)

- **Painkillers:** naproxen (Aleve, Naprosyn), piroxicam (Feldene)

- **Psychiatric drugs:** chlorpromazine (Thorazine), desipramine (Norpramin), imipramine (Tofranil)

possibly damaging the connective tissue that helps maintain the skin's smooth appearance. Cigarette smoking is also associated with a loss of skin elasticity. Plus, smokers suffer much more severe photodamage from sunlight than they would with either smoke or UV radiation by itself. The very worst thing you can do to your skin is to smoke at the beach!

Smoking-related wrinkles may not appear for a decade or more after the first puff, but damage occurs with every cigarette smoked. A study of 79 pairs of identical twins, where only one twin smoked (or smoked at least five years longer than the other), revealed striking differences in their faces. A panel of judges who didn't know which twin was the smoker gave worse scores to the smokers for bags under the eyes, nasolabial folds, upper lip wrinkles, and jowls. Considering how harmful smoking is, not just to your skin but to every other part of your body, the healthiest choice is to avoid cigarettes. If you're trying to quit, support groups, nicotine gum and patches, and the drugs bupropion (Zyban, generic) and varenicline (Chantix, generic) can be useful smoking-cessation tools.

Irritants

Skin becomes thinner and doesn't heal as easily as you age, so take care in handling and working with irritants. Substances that are very acidic or alkaline can damage the skin's top layer and leave it susceptible to infection. You may encounter them on the job in industrial settings where solvents are used. Dust and smoke, such as those from tobacco and wood, and gases, such as mace or tear gas, can damage skin, too. But if you wonder about the kind of irritation caused by vigorous scrubbing of your skin, you can rest easy. Scrubbing generally doesn't damage skin or cause wrinkles. If your skin is irritated by harsh chemicals, apply over-the-counter topical corticosteroids followed by a nonirritating moisturizing cream to help the skin heal. Antibiotics may be needed if infection sets in.

Facial expressions

Laughter may be the best medicine, but there's no getting around the fact that the facial expressions that go with it can add to creases and lines that develop through the years. Facial expressions are an important part of communication; however, every time you smile, squint, or frown, facial muscles contract and cause accordion-like creases to form in your skin. Young skin bounces back. But as aging skin loses its elasticity and firmness, those lines tend to become etched in the skin. Even sleeping with your face scrunched in a pillow at night may cause some lines to gradually appear.

No one would advise you to maintain a stony expression all day to solve this problem. But if you want to go to the trouble, maintaining a pleasant, relaxed facial expression instead of a scowl is a helpful strategy. You can sleep in a position that does not press your face into the pillow. And for those who choose to take further steps, a variety of cosmetic options are available (see "Cosmetic procedures," page 34).

Tanning without the sun

Tanning beds, which expose you to UV radiation, are best avoided altogether. The UV radiation in tanning beds can be 10 to 15 times more powerful than the midday sun. People who frequently go to tanning salons can end up getting 1.2 to 4.7 times the dose that people get from normal sun exposure in a year. That's in addition to any routine sun exposure they get. Regular use of tanning beds increases the risk of melanoma by 74%, as well as the chances of getting basal cell and squamous cell cancers.

If you are concerned about getting enough vitamin D, visiting a tanning salon or soaking up lots of sunshine is not the answer. A very small amount of sun exposure—perhaps five minutes a day, three times a week, to the arms and legs—is sufficient. However, vitamin D from a healthy diet and dietary supplements offer the same benefits as vitamin D obtained from sunlight—without the danger of skin cancer.

If golden skin is important to you, self-tanning and bronzing products are a more effective alternative than they used to be. They no longer turn your skin the color of a pumpkin, and the chemicals appear to be safe when used as directed. Most products use dihydroxyacetone (DHA), a colorless chemical derived from glycerin, which reacts with the amino acids in the outer layers of skin. Thicker, protein-rich areas of your skin will stain more, so for more even results, you should exfoliate the skin of the elbows, knees, and ankles beforehand, using a washcloth, sponge, or loofah, for example. Because the coloring process takes place only in the surface layers of the skin, your "tan" lasts only as long as those layers stay on your body—five to seven days. After they slough off, you'll need a reapplication.

How to do a skin self-exam

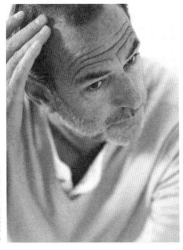

© Goodluz | Thinkstock

To detect skin cancer early, examine your skin all over your body and watch for changes over time. By checking your skin regularly, you'll learn what is normal for you. The best time to check your skin is after a shower or bath. Use a full-length mirror and a hand-held mirror in a room with plenty of light. If you find anything unusual, see your doctor.

Follow these steps to check yourself from head to toe:

1. Look at your face, neck, ears, and scalp. You may want to use a comb or a blow dryer to move your hair so that you can see better. It may be hard to check your scalp by yourself, so you may want to have a relative or friend check through your hair.

2. Look at the front and back of your body in the mirror. Then, raise your arms and look at your left and right sides.

3. Bend your elbows. Look carefully at your fingernails, palms, forearms (including the undersides), and upper arms.

4. Check the back, front, and sides of your legs. Also check the skin all over your buttocks and genital area.

5. Sit and closely examine your feet, including your toenails, the soles of your feet, and the spaces between your toes.

6. Learn where your moles are and their usual look and feel. Check for anything different, such as
   - a new mole (that looks different from your other moles)
   - a new red or darker-colored flaky patch that may be a little raised
   - a change in the size, shape, color, or feel of a mole
   - a sore that doesn't heal
   - a new flesh-colored firm bump.

Write down the dates of your skin self-exams and make notes about the way your skin looks on those dates. You may find it helpful to take photos to help check for changes over time.

Source: National Institutes of Health Senior Health.

Three-step daily skin care

For daily skin care, limit your regimen to three simple steps: cleaning, protecting your skin from the sun, and tending to any specific skin problems you may have such as dry skin, acne, or fine lines and wrinkles. Products for all three steps are available for very little cost at retail stores. Buying expensive skin care lotions with exotic or pseudoscientific names will not produce better results.

1. **Clean your skin.** Choose your skin cleanser based on whether your skin is dry or oily. If you have dry skin, choose a mild cleaning agent (such as Dove, Cetaphil, or Aveeno soaps or cleansers) and avoid products including toners that contain alcohol. For oily skin, choose a soap that removes the oil and cleanse more frequently throughout the day.

2. **Protect your skin from the sun.** Choose a broad-spectrum sunscreen with an SPF of 30 or higher and wear it every day. Higher SPFs are useful if you plan to spend hours outdoors, but if you spend most of your time indoors, SPF 30 is generally sufficient. If you have sensitive skin, choose a sunscreen product designed for sensitive skin.

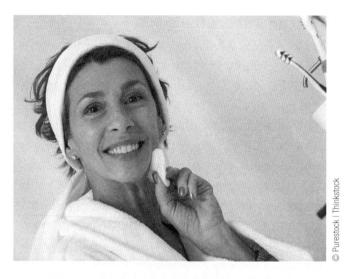

© Purestock | Thinkstock

3. **Treat your particular skin needs.** For dry skin, effective and inexpensive moisturizers are available (see "Dry skin," page 10). For adult acne products, see "Adult acne," page 6. If you want to try a product that moderately reduces lines and wrinkles or fades brown spots, a variety of products that you can use daily are available (see "Cosmeceuticals," page 30).

Manufacturers have also begun adding anti-aging and moisturizing agents, antioxidants, and botanical ingredients to their products, and some allow you to build a tan slowly with repeated applications. Remember, though, that sunless tanners do not protect you from the sun's rays, so be sure to use sunscreen when you're outside.

Self-tanners are available in many forms, including lotions, creams, and sprays that you apply and let soak in to your skin. The FDA cautions users to take care not to get the product in the eyes, nose, or mouth. The FDA has not approved DHA-infused spray-tanning products for use on any part of the body that is covered by a mucous membrane. You should also avoid ingesting sunless tanning products, as the safety of DHA when ingested is unknown.

If you visit a salon that applies such products for you, the FDA recommends first asking these three questions about safety:

- Will my eyes and the area surrounding them be protected?
- Will my nose, mouth, and ears be protected?
- Will I be protected from inhaling the tanning spray through my nose or mouth?

If the answer to any of these questions is "no," look for another salon.

You should also stay away from tanning pills, which are unsafe and can even cause serious health problems. ◗

Lotions and potions

A widely advertised face cream claims to smooth wrinkles with a "patented oligopeptide" for $225 per 1-ounce bottle. Would you buy it? Another lotion claims to allow "deep dermal penetration of nutrients." Do you believe it? These and many other claims for cosmetic products are best viewed with skepticism. Because the FDA doesn't regulate these claims, there often is little or no scientific evidence to back them up. Most cosmetic products will remove more cash from your wallet than wrinkles from your skin.

With the exception of colors and certain prohibited ingredients, a cosmetics manufacturer can use essentially any raw material in a product and market it without FDA approval. This gap in oversight is a cause for concern because of the enormous growth of "cosmeceuticals," chemicals in cosmetics that have physiological effects, such as boosting collagen production and inhibiting sun damage to reduce wrinkles (see "Cosmeceuticals," page 30). A number of cosmeceuticals have actual therapeutic effects, but because they are not classified as drugs, they are exempt from government regulations.

Although cosmetic claims are allowed without scientific substantiation, medical claims, such as removing dandruff or altering skin structure or function, are regulated. A product that makes medical or health claims is classified as a drug for which scientific studies demonstrating safety and effectiveness must be submitted to the FDA.

If you're wondering whether a lotion or cream will do what it claims, understand that only a few substances have a scientifically demonstrated ability to reduce or prevent wrinkles in controlled studies. Such substances are discussed in the following sections. Most of the ingredients in skin care products aren't harmful, but while you may enjoy their fragrance, texture, or temporary effects, think twice about investing too much hope or cash in unproven promises.

Moisturizers

A good moisturizer is one of the foundations of an effective skin care regimen for dry, older skin. Moisturizers can soothe dry skin and make wrinkles less noticeable, even though the effect is temporary. But with so many to choose from, how do you decide?

Petroleum jelly is one of the most effective moisturizers, especially when used right after bathing to seal in moisture (see "Treating dry skin," page 11). It is also one of the least expensive. But many people dislike using it on their faces because it looks and feels greasy. Instead, creams and lotions that contain some water are a better choice for a facial moisturizer. Many of these creams and lotions are humectants, an oil-free class of moisturizer that binds water to skin, so the smoothing, softening effects may last longer.

Most moisturizers contain water, glycerin, petrolatum, stearic acid, propylene glycol, and lanolin. Some contain botanical ingredients, such as jojoba oil, coconut oil, safflower oil, and linoleic acid, which help maintain the skin's outer layer of keratin and keep skin supple. Manufacturers use other ingredients, such as cetyl alcohol, palmitic acid, and dimethicone, to give moisturizers a creamy, velvety, or translucent look and feel, and to help shore up the "mortar" that keeps skin soft and smooth.

fast fact | There are no government standards for the use of words on cosmetic labels such as "natural," "herbal," "dermatologist-tested," "allergy-tested," "nonirritating," "hypoallergenic," or "cruelty-free, non–animal tested." These terms are often employed solely for marketing purposes. The ingredient list on the label is the only source of reliable, government-required information.

Do you need a skin toner?

If your skin has become dry through the years, it may be best to avoid many skin-toning products because they often contain drying, irritating ingredients such as alcohol or acetone. Some also contain highly acidic citrus, camphor, or menthol. However, toners made of water, glycerin, and agents that bind water to the skin offer a bit of extra cleansing and moisture. Skin toners provide no real skin improvement.

Some moisturizers also contain sunscreens and cosmeceuticals, which help prevent or even correct fine wrinkles, uneven skin pigmentation, and other signs of aging and photoaging.

Exfoliants

Moisturizers that contain exfoliant ingredients can improve the appearance of the skin by removing dead surface skin cells. As a result, they can smooth the skin's appearance and even out some discoloration from too much sun exposure. Exfoliants can be particularly useful for aging skin that appears rough and sallow, because older skin doesn't slough off dead surface skin cells as easily as younger skin does.

Two chemical exfoliants, alpha hydroxy acids (AHAs) and beta hydroxy acids (BHAs), are considered superior to many exfoliating scrubs, masks, soaps, toners, and abrasive cloths. That's because they change cell growth patterns and may help renew collagen.

Alpha hydroxy acids

Alpha hydroxy acids (AHAs) are obtained from various fruits, including grapes, citrus fruits, and apples. You'll find them listed on product labels as glycolic acid, lactic acid, malic acid, hydroxycaprylic acid, alpha-hydroxyoctanoic acid, triple fruit acid, or sugar cane extract. Although the FDA does not regulate AHAs as drugs, it has issued guidelines on their safe use because they can cause skin irritation and increase skin sensitivity to UV rays. Choose products that contain an AHA concentration of 10% or less and a pH of 3.5 or more (lower pH numbers are more acidic), and

use a sunscreen in conjunction with AHA-containing products. AHAs, particularly glycolic acid, are used in chemical peels in concentrations of 20% to 30% and higher. An FDA review panel concluded that cosmetologists or skin aestheticians could safely use glycolic acid and lactic acid at concentrations not greater than 30% and with a pH not lower than 3.0 for brief skin care sessions provided that thorough rinsing and daily sun protection follow. In higher concentrations, AHAs should be applied by a physician.

Beta hydroxy acids

Beta hydroxy acids (BHAs), another type of cosmetic exfoliant, are moderately effective at improving the surface of the skin. The BHA used in skin care products is salicylic acid, a relative of aspirin. Salicylic acid is more effective than AHAs in reaching oily areas of the skin such as the pores, which makes it useful if you have oily skin or if you're having problems with acne.

Salicylic acid can be found in many acne products at effective levels of 1.5% to 2%. But antiwrinkle products containing these ingredients tend not to list the percentage on their labels, so it's difficult to know whether they contain sufficient amounts to be effective. The FDA recommends that you first test a BHA product on a small patch of skin to see if irritation occurs, and that you use a sunscreen at the same time because BHA can increase the skin's sun sensitivity.

Cosmeceuticals

Some cosmetics contain ingredients—known in the industry as cosmeceuticals—that have medicinal or druglike benefits. These agents, which include vitamins, growth factors, and peptides, are found in products prescribed by dermatologists and many others that are available over the counter. The FDA does not recognize the term cosmeceutical (nor does it acknowledge the term "skin tightening") and does not regulate most of these substances for safety or effectiveness, although it makes recommendations on some. That means you buy and use cosmetic products at your own risk. Most are safe, but their benefits generally don't live up to the marketing hype that surrounds them.

A few cosmeceuticals show some promise in protecting against the effects of aging and photodamage. Studies demonstrate that they diminish wrinkles and age spots, smooth skin texture, and reduce the yellow hue that comes with age.

Vitamins and antioxidants

Some of the most confusing questions in skin care concern the use of vitamins and antioxidants, such as vitamins A, C, and E and ubiquinone (coenzyme Q_{10}). In theory, the use of these substances in moisturizers and other cosmetics makes sense. At the cellular level, antioxidants ward off damage from molecules called free radicals, which cause oxidative deterioration.

Some vitamins and antioxidants may be beneficial when applied to the skin. Derivatives of vitamin A are the active ingredients in retinoids, drugs that reduce photodamage and increase collagen production (see "Retinoids," at right). Studies have reported that vitamin C helped repair elastic tissue and increase collagen, and that vitamin B_3 (niacinamide) reduced signs of photoaging as well as the cancer-causing effects of ultraviolet radiation. There is limited evidence that coenzyme Q_{10}, a naturally occurring antioxidant, moderately reduces lines and guards against ultraviolet light damage. Alpha lipoic acid, another antioxidant, reportedly decreases wrinkles, age spots, and roughness. Copper, an antioxidant metal, may play a role in collagen and elastin production.

Combining antioxidants may be more effective than using a single antioxidant alone. For example, combining vitamins C and E with ferulic acid, a plant antioxidant, has been shown to help protect against photoaging and skin cancer, as has combining vitamin C, ferulic acid, and phloretin, another antioxidant. Future studies may show new ways of combining antioxidants, applied to the skin or taken as a supplement, to fight wrinkles and prevent sun damage. Regardless of the formulation, antioxidants should be used with sunscreens and retinoids to enhance their protective effects.

Growth factors

Hundreds of growth factors occur naturally in the human body to help heal wounds by promoting new tissue formation. Several studies have found that creams with different combinations of these proteins diminish wrinkles, but more research is needed to confirm these effects. In addition, there are no standards to ensure the quality and stability of products containing growth factors, which can cost upward of $250 per ounce.

Peptides

These compounds, which have various roles in the body, are used as cosmeceuticals for different effects. Some peptides stimulate the production of collagen and elastin. Others stabilize copper (an antioxidant metal shown to reduce wrinkles), improve skin elasticity, and reverse other signs of photoaging. There is some evidence that the peptide dimethylaminoethanol (DMAE), a membrane stabilizer, may firm and smooth skin and decrease wrinkle depth. But more research is needed to confirm the theoretical benefits of these compounds.

Retinoids

Topical vitamin A–based drugs called retinoids—the most used and most studied anti-aging compounds—may reduce fine lines and wrinkles. Tretinoin, under the brand name Retin-A, was the first retinoid. It was used as an acne treatment in the 1970s, but researchers later discovered that it also fades actinic keratosis spots, evens pigmentation, and speeds the turnover of superficial skin cells.

Retinoids reduce fine lines and wrinkles by increasing the production of collagen. They also stimulate the production of new blood vessels in the skin, which improves skin color. Additional benefits include fading age spots and softening rough patches of skin. However, it takes three to six months of regular use before improvements in wrinkles are apparent—and the best results take six to 12 months. Because retinoids can cause skin dryness and irritation, doctors often recommend using them only every other day at first and then gradually working up to nightly applications. Wear a sunscreen during the day, because retinoids increase the skin's sensitivity to sunlight. These drugs must be used continually to maintain their benefits.

Quick guide to product ingredients

The labels of anti-aging products promote some impressive-sounding ingredients. What are they? Can they help your skin? This glossary defines many of the terms or ingredient names you are likely to encounter. But keep in mind that most cosmetic products are not regulated, and in most cases there is little or no published evidence to substantiate their effectiveness.

- **Alpha lipoic acid:** An antioxidant claimed to have a modest effect in decreasing skin roughness and wrinkles.

- **Antioxidants:** Substances that neutralize free radicals, damaging molecules that accelerate cellular aging and promote cancer.

- **Coenzyme Q10:** Ubiquinone, an antioxidant that protects against UVA and may modestly reduce wrinkle depth.

- **Copper peptide:** Copper is a metal with antioxidant properties found in every cell in the human body. Copper peptides (see "Peptides," below) enhance wound healing and may modestly increase collagen and elastin production.

- **Dimethylaminoethanol (DMAE):** A neurotransmitter produced in the brain; an extract in gel form is purported to reduce wrinkles, neck sagging, and circles under the eyes.

- **Genistein:** A derivative of soy and an antioxidant; it inhibits UVB damage to the skin.

- **Green tea:** An antioxidant and an anti-inflammatory agent; it may inhibit UV damage and photoaging.

- **Growth factors:** Substances that occur naturally in the human body and in plants; they contribute to wound healing and may repair photodamaged skin.

- **Kinetin:** N6-furfuryladenine; a plant growth factor and an antioxidant claimed to reduce wrinkles, smooth skin texture, and even out skin tone.

- **Niacinamide:** Vitamin B_3; an antioxidant that is promoted to help reverse signs of photoaging.

- **Peptides:** Short-chain amino acids that may assist with production of collagen and elastin or have other beneficial effects on the skin.

- **Retinoid:** Any of several derivatives of vitamin A that have been shown to reduce photodamage and increase collagen production.

- **Vitamin C (ascorbic acid):** In topical preparations, it is thought to reduce wrinkles and improve skin texture and tone.

- **Vitamin E:** An antioxidant vitamin; limited research suggests some protective effects for the skin.

Tretinoin (Retin-A, generic), tazarotene (Avage, Tazorac), and adapalene (Differin) are prescription retinoids. Adapalene is also available over the counter (in a 0.1% formulation versus the 0.3% prescription version). Other retinoids are undergoing clinical trials.

In addition, several over-the-counter products containing retinoids, such as retinol, are available. Because they're not as strong (and thus less irritating), they are not as effective in reducing wrinkles as tretinoin, but they do improve the appearance of photoaged skin. Tretinoin can be used with AHAs for additional skin-smoothing effects.

Other skin care products

Thousands of products and substances are currently being marketed for skin enhancement. Here are three common categories:

Muds and other mineral products. Salts, muds, and clays are often purported to have natural minerals that restore youthful softness and luster to your skin. While some of these products may leave your skin with a nice clean feel or smell, it is important to recognize that the molecules in them are generally too large to penetrate the skin. In most cases, there are no published scientific data to back up their claims.

Products from plant sources. Some plants have bioactive properties. Lotions and creams with extracts from plants, such as aloe, seaweed, fruits, or herbs, can contain any number of other ingredients that have a variety of effects on the skin. Aloe vera gel, which is extracted from the fleshy leaves of the aloe vera plant, is commonly used for burns, sunburn, frostbite, psoriasis, and cold sores. In addition to AHAs, some other plant-based ingredients, such as soy, mushroom, and feverfew, may reduce or prevent wrinkles, but so far the evidence comes from small studies and animal research. Many other plant-based products have a pleasant scent and come attractively packaged. Plant-based products are generally safe to use topically, but you should understand that there is little evidence regarding their effectiveness. Also, watch for any skin reaction, as some may cause allergies in some people.

Masks. Hydrating and firming sheet masks have become very popular in recent years, in addition to applied masks. They contain a variety of compounds, including botanicals and hyaluronic acid, that may or may not be beneficial to the skin—but typically do leave it appearing better, at least temporarily.

What to avoid

It's always important to read the ingredient labels of creams and lotions, especially if you have sensitive skin. Although irritation from moisturizers is uncommon, some products may contain substances that can cause problems. The American Academy of Dermatology advises people with sensitive skin to avoid skin care products with the following ingredients:

Fragrances and preservatives. Many fragrances and preservatives can irritate skin. If possible, use products without them. The least irritating preservatives are parabens, such as methyl paraben and butyl paraben. These preservatives have been used for more than 80 years and appear to be safe and well tolerated. But parabens bind with human estrogen receptors (although very weakly), and research suggesting possible associations with decreased sperm quality and breast cancer has sparked concern about the chemicals. Because of customer concerns, many manufacturers have removed them from products, although other studies haven't confirmed the worrisome findings. While further study is warranted, the current evidence doesn't support a need to restrict exposure.

Botanical or antibacterial ingredients. "Natural" ingredients aren't always benign. If you have allergies or sensitive skin, you may find that plant extracts cause a reaction. Antibacterial lotions can also be irritating for some people.

Solvents. Chemicals that penetrate the skin include propylene glycol and ethanol. A better alternative is polyethylene glycol, which does not penetrate the skin. ▼

Cosmetic procedures

If Ponce de Leon returned today to search for the fountain of youth, he might find that the secret to youthful skin lies in powerful lasers, injectable wrinkle fillers, and other recent technologies that can remove fine lines, fill in deeper ones, and lighten unsightly pigmented areas or spots. These procedures help rejuvenate skin worn by time and sun exposure, with few side effects and far less recovery time than that required for surgical techniques such as facelifts.

Recovery time—the time it takes for skin to heal and return to normal color and texture—is one of the most important factors for people seeking such cosmetic procedures. Most people want to return to work and social activities as quickly as possible, which has led to the increased use of less invasive techniques that don't wound the skin as extensively as the deep chemical peels and full laser resurfacing that used to predominate. The trade-off is that their effects are not as significant, and they often require a series of treatments as well as follow-up "maintenance" visits. How-ever, with today's more sophisticated laser treatments, it is now possible to find a happy medium: moderate effects with minimal downtime.

The techniques described in this chapter fall into four general categories:
- injectable treatments that smooth and fill wrinkles
- skin resurfacing techniques that target fine lines, age spots, and skin discoloration
- skin tightening or lifting procedures that smooth and tone skin, especially around the eyes, jaw, and neckline
- light-based treatments using LED or other lights to tone the skin.

These techniques may be used alone, but increasingly they are used in combination, or with other cosmetic techniques, to treat deeper wrinkles or scars on one area of the face and finer lines or superficial lesions on another. Clinicians often recommend a combination of procedures to achieve a desired effect. For example, for an older woman seeking more pro-

At what age is it best to begin cosmetic treatment?

Dermatologists are often asked at what age a person who wants cosmetic treatments should start. There are no hard-and-fast rules, but some procedures tend to be used more at certain times of life than others—and many experts say it is never too early for adults to begin.

Many dermatologists believe that neuromodulator treatments such as botulinum toxin should be started between the ages of 20 and 30. The frown lines and crow's feet that develop over the years are a result of your facial expressions. By diminishing the movement of the muscles that cause those expressions, neuromodulators effectively prevent the lines from forming in the first place.

Doctors tend to recommend soft-tissue fillers in midlife and beyond, to plump up folds and sunken areas in the face. But these, too, have a role in preventing further deterioration of your appearance. Studies suggest that filler injections stimulate the body's own natural collagen production, and dermatologists say that the more filler a person uses, the less often repeat injections are needed (and, over time, they become unnecessary).

For facelifts, most doctors now recommend getting a series of small, subtle facelifts starting in middle age rather than waiting for a major facelift later in life.

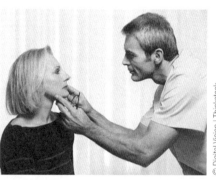

© Digital Vision | Thinkstock

Similarly, with respect to laser and light-based treatments, one study found that a series of three broadband light treatments actually altered gene expression in aging skin, so that it behaved more like younger skin. For those with fair skin in particular, it makes sense to start in the 30s and 40s when changes in skin become apparent.

nounced skin tightening and who is willing to put up with some downtime, a doctor might recommend botulinum toxin for frown lines and forehead lines, fillers for nasolabial folds, Q-switched laser or intense pulsed light treatments to remove freckling and diminish redness, plus fractional laser resurfacing for all-over improvement. Table 2 lists the most common problems and available treatments; the rest of this chapter describes the therapies in greater detail.

Just remember: While these treatments are getting better all the time, the goal is improvement, not perfection—and skin continues aging, whether you treat it or not, so no single procedure will restore youthful skin for good.

Doctor or aesthetician?

Some procedures that affect only superficial layers of skin can be performed by nurses or skin aestheticians, while others require the skills of a dermatologist or other physician. Whom you trust to perform a procedure is a crucial factor in whether the outcome will be successful.

While less invasive procedures such as microdermabrasion can be performed by cosmetology professionals, skin surgeries, including laser procedures, should be performed by physicians from a number of specialties: dermatologists and dermatologic surgeons, plastic surgeons, facial plastic surgeons (otolaryngologists), oculoplastic surgeons (ophthalmologists), and other cosmetic surgeons. In some settings, nurses or physician assistants with special training may perform some of these procedures. Beware of laser and filler treatments at "medspas" that are performed by technicians with minimal training.

Choosing a doctor or other skin specialist

One way to start is with a dermatologist who can advise you about which procedures are best handled by a physician. Some physicians who perform cosmetic procedures also have nurses or aestheticians or both on staff to handle the less invasive treatments.

To find a reputable physician, begin by asking your own doctor for recommendations. Or contact professional societies that have sophisticated referral ser-

Questions to ask the doctor

Before undergoing any cosmetic procedure that requires a medical professional, such as botulinum toxin injections, filler injections, or laser resurfacing, ask how many procedures of this type the clinician performs per month or year. Also find out how long he or she has been doing this procedure, and whether he or she has written about or taught the procedure in an academic setting. Expertise levels can vary, but you want someone who has had specialized training, perhaps a fellowship in an academic medical center, rather than just a course or two. How many procedures of any kind does the clinician perform per day? You don't want a surgeon who is rushed or who won't give you full, personal attention.

You should also ask about cost. For example, is there a consultation fee, and if so, can it be deducted from the cost of the procedure? What is the complete cost for the procedure, including the physician's fee, anesthesiology, and operating room costs? Who delivers the anesthesia? Ask if the clinician charges extra for corrections or repairs, and make sure you understand the complications that could occur and exactly what is involved in recovery. The healing process for some procedures can be lengthy and tedious. Another important consideration is whether the procedure will need to be repeated and how often. Some of the less invasive procedures have shorter recovery times, but require several treatments or even periodic maintenance procedures every few months.

And don't forget to trust your gut. Choose a physician with whom you feel comfortable and can establish an easy rapport. It's helpful, too, if the physician has a courteous, knowledgeable staff. Finally, keep in mind that no matter how talented or experienced your physician is, no amount of filling, lasering, or peeling is going to make you look 20 years old again.

vices and websites with information about physicians' training and experience, the articles they've written, and the procedures they perform (see "Resources," page 51). In some areas, city or county medical associations can provide names of local physicians.

You can also ask friends, co-workers, or family members who've had cosmetic procedures if they were satisfied with the results and whether they would go back to the same physician. But remember that doctors who are popular or who advertise heavily may not be highly skilled, or they may not be right for you.

Once you have the name of a physician, the next step is to check whether he or she is board-certified. Many consumers know to ask about certification, but might not ask which board has done the certifying, or

Table 2: Common cosmetic problems and their treatments

Depending on the cosmetic problem you wish to solve, a range of nonsurgical options are available. You'll need to evaluate the choices based on their effectiveness, cost, recovery time, safety, and other factors. Repeat treatments are necessary for most of these procedures in order to attain the desired effect or to maintain the results over the long term.

PROBLEM	TREATMENT CHOICES	EFFECTIVENESS	COMMENTS
Entire face			
Brown spots on face or hands	Bleaching creams	Mildly effective	Inexpensive. Safe. No recovery time. Many applications needed to produce only a mild effect.
	Retinoid creams	Moderately effective	Moderately expensive. Will lighten but not fully remove brown spots. Can cause skin irritation. May be combined with bleaching creams.
	Chemical peels	Moderately effective	Expensive. Recovery time depends on strength of peel solution.
	Fractional non-ablative laser resurfacing (Clear + Brilliant, Fraxel DUAL, Fraxel re:store, Palomar Lux 1540)	Effective	Expensive. Short recovery time (swelling, 3–5 days).
	Pulsed light therapy (Cutera Xeo, Icon)	Very effective	Expensive. Short recovery time (3–5 days). May cause redness or swelling for a few days; brown spots will dry up and flake off for 7–10 days.
	Q-switched laser	Very effective	Expensive. Moderate recovery time (crusts, 7–10 days).
Red skin or veins	Vasoconstricting creams and gels (for rosacea) such as brimonidine gel (Mirvaso)	Effective	Inexpensive. Reduces redness for approximately eight hours. May make some people too pale.
	Pulsed dye laser (yellow light) or pulsed Nd:YAG laser (green light)	Very effective	Expensive. Moderate recovery time; bruising possible.
	Pulsed light therapy (Cutera Xeo, Icon)	Very effective	Expensive. Moderate recovery time. Causes temporary redness and occasionally some swelling for a few days if large areas are treated.
Fine lines or fine wrinkles	Lotions containing alpha hydroxy acids or beta hydroxy acids	Mildly effective	Inexpensive products are available without prescription.
	Growth factors	Moderately effective	Expensive. No recovery time.
	Microneedling (Collagen P.I.N., DermaFrac, Dermapen, Eclipse MicroPen, Juvapen, SkinPen)	Moderately effective	Moderately expensive. May leave skin red or puffy for a couple of days. A series of two to three treatments spaced six to eight weeks apart is typically recommended.
	Microdermabrasion	Moderately effective	Moderately expensive. No recovery time, but may cause some temporary pinkness.
	Chemical peels	Moderately effective to effective	Expensive. Recovery time depends on the choice and strength of the peel solution.
	Fractional non-ablative laser resurfacing (Clear + Brilliant, Fraxel DUAL, Fraxel re:store, Palomar Lux 1540)	Effective	Expensive. Short recovery time.
	Retinoid creams	Effective	Lower-strength products available without prescription. More expensive, stronger products available with prescription.

continued on page 37

Table 2 *continued*

PROBLEM	TREATMENT CHOICES	EFFECTIVENESS	COMMENTS
Fine lines or fine wrinkles *(continued)*	Fractional ablative laser resurfacing (Active FX, Deep FX, Fraxel re:pair SST, SmartXide DOX)	Very effective	Very expensive. Moderate recovery time. Longer recovery than fractional non-ablative laser resurfacing but fewer treatments needed.
Forehead lines	Botulinum toxin injections (Botox, Dysport, Xeomin)	Very effective	Expensive. Repeat treatments necessary. No recovery time.
	Injectable fillers (Belatero, Juvaderm Ultra, Juvederm Vobella XC, Restylane)	Very effective	Expensive. Short recovery time; bruising possible. Used less commonly than botulinum toxin, but can be combined with botulinum toxin.
Unwanted hair	Electrolysis	Moderately effective	Expensive. Removes both dark and light hair. Painful. Can treat only limited areas at one visit. Takes many treatments.
	Pulsed light therapy (Cutera Xeo, Icon)	Moderately effective	Expensive. Removes dark hair only. Cannot be used on dark or tanned skin. Takes many treatments.
	Laser removal (Apogee, GentleLase, GentleYAG, LightSheer Duet Diode, Profile)	Very effective	Expensive. Removes dark hair only. Painful. Takes many treatments. Can treat large areas at one time.

Around the eyes

Lines around eyes	Fractional non-ablative laser resurfacing (Clear + Brilliant, Fraxel DUAL, Fraxel re:store, Palomar Lux 1540)	Mildly effective for fine lines	Very expensive. Longer lasting. Short recovery time.
	Botulinum toxin injections (Botox, Dysport, Xeomin)	Very effective for expression lines	Expensive. Repeat treatments necessary. No recovery time.
	Fractional ablative laser resurfacing (Active FX, Deep FX, Fraxel re:pair SST, SmartXide DOX)	Very effective	Very expensive. Up to a week-long recovery time.
Undereye wrinkles, bags, or crepey skin	Creams and gels	Mildly effective	Inexpensive to moderately expensive. No recovery time.
	Radiofrequency treatment (Aluma, Elos, Pellevé, Thermage)	Moderately effective	Expensive. No recovery time.
	Fractional ablative laser resurfacing (Active FX, Deep FX, Fraxel re:pair SST, SmartXide DOX)	Very effective	Very expensive. Up to a week-long recovery time.

Lower face and neck

Nasolabial folds	Injectable fillers (Belatero, Bellafill, Juvaderm Ultra, Juvaderm Ultra Plus, Radiesse, Restylane, Restylane Lyft, Sculptra, Voluma, autologous fat)	Very effective	Expensive. Occasional bruising. Short recovery time. Slight risk of lumps. Repeat treatments may be necessary.
Double chin	Cryolipolysis (Cool Mini)	Very effective	Expensive. One-hour treatment. Can be done more than once.
	Injections (Kybella)	Very effective	Expensive. Requires 10 to 15 injection sites and topical or local anesthesia. May cause swelling for one week. Treatment is often repeated two or three times.

continued on page 37

Table 2 *continued*

PROBLEM	TREATMENT CHOICES	EFFECTIVENESS	COMMENTS
Sagging neck skin	Botulinum toxin injections (Botox, Dysport, Xeomin)	Effective for neck cords	Expensive.
	Focused ultrasound skin tightening (Ulthera)	Moderately effective	Expensive. Moderately painful.
	External radiofrequency skin tightening (Aluma, Elos, Pellevé, Thermage)	Moderately effective	Expensive. Not painful. No recovery time.
	Fractional non-ablative laser resurfacing (Clear + Brilliant, Fraxel DUAL, Fraxel re:store, Palomar Lux 1540)	Moderately effective	Expensive. Short recovery time.
	Internal radiofrequency-induced skin tightening (ThermiTight)	Very effective	Expensive. Minimal discomfort. Usually just one treatment is needed.
	Fractional high-intensity focused radiofrequency (Endymed Intensif, Infini)	Very effective	Expensive. Three treatments ae typically needed.
	Fractional ablative laser resurfacing (Active FX, Deep FX, Fraxel re:pair SST, SmartXide DOX)	Very effective	Very expensive. Slightly longer recovery but fewer treatments needed. Some risks.
Jaw line droop	Radiofrequency skin tightening (Aluma, Elos, Pellevé, Thermage)	Moderately effective	Expensive. Not painful. No recovery time. Results may be subtle.
	Focused ultrasound (Ulthera)	Moderately effective	Expensive. Painful.

whether that board is overseen by the American Board of Medical Specialties (ABMS). The ABMS oversees 24 approved medical specialty boards in the United States. A number of other groups may call themselves "boards," but they aren't overseen by the ABMS. Their certification requirements may be less rigorous than boards that are under ABMS purview. More than 100 of these self-designated boards exist throughout the United States, and there are virtually no legal requirements for their formation. Some may be no more than glorified public relations offices. To check qualifications, contact the ABMS's Doctor Verification Service toll-free at 866-275-2267, or online at www.abms.org.

The American Board of Dermatology, a founding member of the ABMS, certifies physicians to perform both general and specialty dermatologic care. Some dermatologists pursue an additional year or two of training to specialize in dermatologic surgery.

The American Board of Plastic Surgery, which is also overseen by the ABMS, certifies physicians to perform the complete array of cosmetic and reconstructive surgical procedures. Physicians certified by this board have a medical degree from an accredited institution, at least two years of residency training in general surgery, and at least two years of additional training in plastic surgery.

If you're going to have a surgical procedure in the physician's office, ask if the office is accredited by one of the following organizations: the American Association for Accreditation of Ambulatory Surgery Facilities, the Accreditation Association for Ambulatory Health Care, or the Joint Commission. Most of the organizations listed in the Resources section of this report (see page 51) offer referral services and can give you the names of physicians in your area.

Choosing an aesthetician

Professional training in nonmedical skin care used to come under the umbrella of cosmetology. Anyone who wanted to specialize in skin care also had to learn how to cut, color, and style hair and how to do nails. Today, though, the health and medical aspects of skin care are recognized with specialized aesthetician (or esthetician) training and licensing.

Aestheticians perform a variety of skin care procedures—deep cleansing, facials, low-grade chemical peels, and microdermabrasion. (True dermabrasion should be performed only by an experienced physician.) While most aestheticians work in salons and spas, don't be surprised if your dermatologist or cosmetic surgeon has an aesthetician on staff. In addition to performing noninvasive treatments, an aesthetician may assist your doctor in pre- and post-procedure skin care and teach you makeup techniques to cover redness or scars.

Licensing requirements for aestheticians vary from state to state, ranging from 250 to 1,000 hours, with an average of 600 hours of classroom time and supervised time treating patients. Contact your state's department of licensing and regulation to learn about licensing requirements in your area. Many states offer this information online.

Most of the techniques described in this section are available at both dermatologists' offices and "medspas"—nonmedical facilities that offer a range of cosmetic services. However, in some spas and similar offices, people who are not well trained do some of the treatments—which can be dangerous. A study published in *JAMA Dermatology* found that the percentage of lawsuits from skin laser surgery performed by nonphysicians more than doubled from 2008 to 2011, calling into question the safety of some medspas. If you do decide to see an aesthetician instead of a dermatologist, make sure the practitioner is licensed in your state and is certified by the National Coalition of Estheticians, Manufacturers/Distributors and Associations (NCEA).

Injectable treatments

These therapies treat small lines and age-associated wrinkles, as well as deeper wrinkles and larger nasolabial folds.

Botulinum toxin

Since botulinum toxin injections were first used for cosmetic purposes in the late 1980s, this therapy has gained quite a following. According to the American Society for Aesthetic Plastic Surgery, in 2015 (the last year for which complete data are available), providers delivered about 4.3 million botulinum toxin injections, making it one of the leading nonsurgical cosmetic procedures in the United States among both sexes and all age groups. In addition to Botox, the best-known brand, there are now two other brands of botulinum toxin injections—Dysport and Xeomin. Other botulinum toxin products with longer-lasting

---

Figure 4: Down with the frown

● = Injection sites

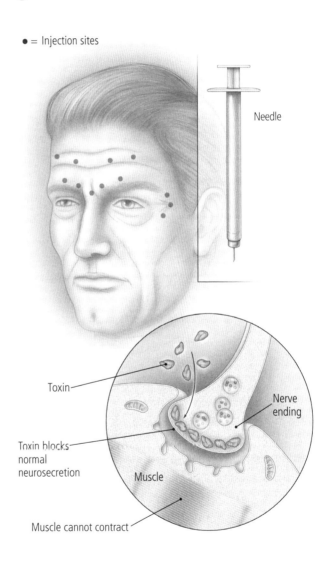

An injection of botulinum toxin can eliminate deeper lines and wrinkles around the forehead, between the eyebrows, at the corner of the eyes, and other locations. Botulinum toxin works by blocking the release of the neurotransmitter acetylcholine, which helps trigger muscle movement, from nerve cells. Impairing the muscle movement allows the creases in the skin to smooth out and prevents the formation of new expression lines.

effects are currently undergoing clinical trials.

Why is this treatment for wrinkles and frown lines so popular? Botulinum toxin injections are relatively affordable, averaging $317 per treatment; have very few risks; and require no recovery time. And they're quite effective at temporarily smoothing a wrinkled face, brow, or neck. Effects generally last three to four months. With continued use, the effects tend to last longer, and the therapy inhibits the formation of deeper, more permanent facial lines over time.

Botulinum toxin type A is a protein produced by the bacterium *Clostridium botulinum*. If you ingest this bacterium in improperly preserved foods or if it infects a wound, it can cause botulism, a rare but potentially deadly disease. But when tiny doses of sterile, purified botulinum toxin are injected into specific muscle sites, the solution doesn't enter the bloodstream, and the procedure causes no harm. The amount used in a cosmetic treatment is far less than the amount necessary to cause illness.

Botulinum toxin works by blocking the release of the neurotransmitter acetylcholine, which helps trigger muscle movement (see Figure 4). By blocking acetylcholine in a few strategic areas, botulinum toxin interferes with the ability of the selected muscles to contract, effectively immobilizing them. The muscles controlling facial expressions relax, and creases in the skin smooth out. Because the muscle can't contract, new creases don't form.

Botulinum toxin injections take just minutes and don't cause much discomfort. You may notice mild redness for a few hours, a minor headache, or occasionally minor bruising, which you can camouflage with makeup. You should notice a change in your appearance in three to seven days.

Many people worry that botulinum toxin injections will leave them with an unnatural expression or with frozen or asymmetrical features. But when done well, botulinum toxin injections shouldn't drastically change your ability to form facial expressions. In rare cases, injections near the upper eyelids or eyebrows may make them droop temporarily. But side effects are typically uncommon and minimal.

However, safety with botulinum toxin is a real concern when poorly trained, unlicensed practitioners deliver it. Experts warn that a "Botox party" in someone's home or office is not an appropriate or safe way to receive a medical treatment, even a cosmetic one. Also beware of Internet sites selling botulinum toxin from unknown locations. These may be bogus products or simply a hoax to take your money.

Botulinum toxin acts on dynamic wrinkles: the lines etched by facial expressions such as laughing, smiling, frowning, wincing, squinting, and pursing your lips. It does not effectively treat the deep creases from nose to mouth known as nasolabial folds. And sometimes a dynamic scowl line is too deep and entrenched to relax. In these cases, you may also need soft-tissue fillers (see below) to raise the depressed surface area left by the lines. Botulinum toxin also doesn't improve the appearance of static wrinkles, which form because of photoaging or chronological aging. Laser resurfacing does a better job on those.

Botulinum toxin is often used along with other cosmetic procedures. Doctors sometimes recommend it with laser resurfacing, since skin heals better when it's not in constant motion, or to enhance results with soft-tissue augmentation. Botulinum toxin injections should be continued after a facelift or skin resurfacing, keeping the newly smooth face and skin from becoming creased again.

Soft-tissue fillers

Soft-tissue fillers are injected under the skin to add height to cheekbones, improve the jaw line, diminish acne or surgical scars, restore fullness to hollow cheeks and eyes, fill vertical fine lines, and resculpt lips that have been thinned by sun exposure or smoking. They can also fill in nasolabial folds, the deep lines that run from the outside of the nostrils to the corners of the mouth that virtually no other skin rejuvenation procedure can correct. This technique minimizes deep lines, wrinkles, and grooves by lifting the surrounding skin and concealing surface imperfections. Fillers are both beauty enhancers and buffers against telltale signs of aging.

With aging, many people lose collagen and fat under the skin. This process is called soft-tissue atrophy. Soft-tissue loss commonly affects the lips and corners of the mouth, the chin, the cheeks, the areas

Choosing a soft-tissue filler

When choosing a filler, consider the area you're having filled. For instance, using fat to fill an area that once had fat, such as the cheeks, can give that area a natural look. But fat may not take as well in areas that have very little fat, such as the forehead. You should also take into account your doctor's expertise with a particular material. Different fillers require different techniques and may be difficult to use correctly, leading to bruising or unwanted results. The following are the mostly commonly used types:

Hyaluronic acid (Belatero, Juvaderm Ultra, Juvaderm Ultra Plus, Restylane, Restylane Lyft, Voluma, others). Hyaluronic acid is a sugar found in numerous tissues, including the skin and cartilage. In the skin, hyaluronic acid is the natural cushion that occupies the spaces between the collagen and elastin fibers, adding bulk (volume) to the skin's dermis. Most of these products, which are the most commonly used fillers, are produced for medical purposes from bacteria. Because the substance is the same from species to species, it carries little risk of allergic reactions. Another advantage is that the volumizing effects are reversible; if you're not happy with the way you look, your doctor can inject an enzyme called hyaluronidase to break down the hyaluronic acid.

Thinner solutions treat finer lines and wrinkles such as crow's feet, while thicker, more viscous gels fill in deeper nasolabial folds, add volume to the face, and make the lips fuller. Hyaluronic acid fillers last longest in the areas of the face that move the least—six months to a year in the cheeks or below the eyes and three to four months in the lips. After subsequent injections they last a lot longer. A second injection, for example, may last a year. Rare side effects include red or swollen small bumps that usually disappear over time.

Poly-L-lactic acid (Sculptra). This substance, which is gradually absorbed by the body, has been used for decades in dissolvable stitches. The FDA approved Sculptra for treating facial fat loss or wasting seen in people with HIV/AIDS in 2004 and for cosmetic purposes (mostly for plumping smile lines and marionette lines, as well as adding cheek volume) in 2009. It stimulates collagen production and lasts up to two years. Side effects include injection site discomfort, redness, bruising, bleeding, itching, and swelling. Small lumps felt under the skin are also possible, as are larger lumps that may be inflamed or discolored.

Microsphere-based fillers (Bellafill, Radiesse). Microspheres are tiny, round particles of solid material. Successful use of these synthetic, longer-lasting injectables depends on the technique used and the skill of the physician. Radiesse is a combination of gel and particles made of calcium hydroxylapatite, a substance found in teeth and bone that is also used as a bone cement. As a filler, it provides a scaffolding for cells that make collagen. The material usually lasts for a year or more. Bellafill is a gel that contains polymethylmethacrylate (plastic) microspheres suspended in bovine collagen. The body absorbs the collagen, and the beads are engulfed by your own collagen to form a lasting implant that lifts lines, wrinkles, scars, and atrophic areas. The beads are not metabolized by the body, and the results may be permanent. Aside from uncommon allergic reactions to bovine collagen, side effects may include inflammation and small bumps in the skin. Both of these products can cause redness, bruising, swelling, and itching.

Silicone (AdatoSil 5000, Silikon 1000). Like Bellafill, silicone is a permanent filler to plump up the volume of the skin and lips and fill in wrinkles and acne scars. The brands mentioned here are approved by the FDA for treating retinal detachment in the eye, but are used off-label for cosmetic purposes. Side effects occur rarely, but the results aren't reversible, so it's advisable to try one of the temporary fillers listed above first to see how you like the results before you commit to a permanent change.

Body fat. In a procedure called an autologous fat transplant, the physician extracts some of your own fat from your hip, thigh, abdomen, or buttock, and then injects it to fill lines or contour hollow areas of your face. Most people have a touch-up in three or four months; your doctor can freeze some of the extracted fat for this purpose. After the second treatment, many people find that results will last five to 10 years.

In many ways, fat is an ideal filler. It's readily available, easy to get, and inexpensive. And if it comes from your own body, it won't cause an immune reaction. Once implanted, it stays in place and is extremely long-lasting. It works best when injected into another fat-containing site, such as areas around the nose and mouth, cheeks, cheekbones, or jaw line. Using fat is more complex and expensive than other procedures, however, and other filler options have become more readily available, so doctors and patients are choosing fat transplants less frequently than in the past.

---

under and between the eyes, and the nasolabial folds. As these areas become less plump, they fold more easily. Injections of soft-tissue fillers can often remedy this. These procedures are popular because they can accentuate the positive and minimize the negative in your face. They aren't as invasive or costly as a facelift, and they don't require much recovery time.

Injectable fillers come in many different concentrations and formulations, depending on the depth of lines and wrinkles to remedy (see "Choosing a soft-tissue filler," above). With so many old and new selections available, deciding which filler might suit your needs has become a complicated process. Do you want something temporary that has a very low risk, or would you prefer something more permanent, even if it has a higher complication rate? Are you willing to try a new product, or do you want something that has a proven track record?

You'll likely receive injections at several sites. Usually, the doctor inserts tiny amounts in the skin, carefully layering the material up to the desired fullness. He or she then gently massages the area to spread the material evenly. A session typically takes 15 to 30 minutes, and costs vary with the material used, ranging from about $600 to $800. You'll need little follow-up care, other than ice during the first few hours.

If you are considering a soft-tissue filler, you should make sure you are comfortable with the procedure. Here are some questions to ask your doctor:

- How long have you used this product or technique? How often do you use it?
- How widely used is this product? If it is new or uncommon, is it substantially better for my needs than other products?
- What material is the filler or implant? Is it natural or synthetic?
- How often do you see complications or side effects?

- Are the results of the treatment temporary, long-lasting, or permanent?
- If the procedure is permanent, can I have it modified or removed?

Fat-dissolving treatments for a double chin

Many people are bothered by double chins and try to conceal them behind turtleneck shirts and scarves. However, recent advancements have expanded the options for jowl removal beyond surgery to in-office treatments.

Cryolipolysis (Cool Mini)

This procedure, also known as "cool sculpting," treats a double chin. The clinician places a handpiece under the chin and chills fat cells there almost to the point of freezing, damaging their membranes so they are absorbed and metabolized by the body. The treatment itself takes about an hour, and results are seen over the subsequent two months. The procedure is quite effective and can be performed more than once. It can also be used to reduce love handles on the waist. The cost is approximately $1,000 per treatment.

Table 3: The 5 most popular nonsurgical cosmetic procedures

More than 13.5 million cosmetic procedures were performed in the United States at a cost of $13.5 billion in 2015 (the last year for which complete data are available). Most were nonsurgical procedures; the most common of these appear below.

PROCEDURE	NUMBER PERFORMED	AVERAGE LENGTH OF PROCEDURE	AVERAGE NUMBER OF PROCEDURES	AVERAGE PRICE*
Botulinum toxin injection	4.3 million	30 minutes	Repeat treatments every three to four months	$317
Hyaluronic acid filler injection	2.1 million	Less than one hour	Repeat treatments every six to 12 months	$591
Laser or pulsed light hair removal	1.1 million	One to two hours, depending on area	Multiple sessions	$254
Chemical peel	603,000	One-half to three hours	One or multiple sessions (depending on type)	$628
Microdermabrasion	558,000	One-half to one hour	Multiple sessions, two- to three-week intervals	$129

*Average prices reflect the doctor's (or other provider's) fees for a procedure performed once and on one site only. For procedures performed on more than one site, the total cost will depend on the number of sites.
Source: American Society for Aesthetic Plastic Surgery, 2015.

Injections to damage fat (Kybella)

This product, approved by the FDA in 2016, contains a substance that damages fat cells. After applying local or topical anesthesia, the physician selects 10 to 15 injection sites in the neck area. The shots can be slightly uncomfortable, and there is potential for swelling, pain, and redness for one week. The fat under the chin will disappear over the course of the next four to six weeks. Like cryolipolysis, these injections are very effective and can be repeated two or three times. The cost is similar, too: about $1,000.

Skin resurfacing

These techniques use different strategies, including chemicals that dissolve skin cells, tools that gently polish the skin's surface, and targeted, intense beams of light (lasers) to improve the skin's appearance.

Chemical peels

Once the first choice for facial rejuvenation, photodamage, fine lines, and pigmentation, chemical peels now play second fiddle to newer, less invasive techniques, but still have a significant role. Peels are used to treat wrinkles, age spots, discoloration, precancerous skin growths, and superficial scarring. An acid solution is applied to the skin, dissolving skin cells and removing the top layers of the epidermis. Just how deeply the peel penetrates, and the effects, vary depending on the type and strength of the solution used. Chemical peels can be done on the hands as well as the face. There is an abundance of research supporting the usefulness of these treatments, which can be done in a doctor's office or a salon.

Recovery time also varies, as some solutions may leave only mild redness for a few days while others produce more extreme redness and peeling that needs to be carefully bandaged and takes weeks to heal.

The most commonly used cosmetic peels contain glycolic or salicylic acid. These mild peels have no permanent effects on the skin, but temporarily improve its appearance and texture and can be repeated intermittently.

For more advanced sun damage or if you want a more noticeable improvement to mild wrinkles, skin tone, and coloring, you may consider a stronger therapeutic peel. These peels dissolve the skin into the top layer of dermis and require a longer recovery time. A solution of 35% to 50% trichloroacetic acid (TCA) is commonly used. Afterward, you'll have mild discomfort, and a few days to a week after the treatment, the superficial skin will darken, turn stiff, and peel off. Your skin may appear flushed for several weeks. Results last up to two years, but many people repeat the treatment annually.

Side effects of chemical peels include redness, itching, peeling, increased skin sensitivity, altered pigmentation, and sometimes fragile and blistering skin. Allergic contact dermatitis can occur, and if your peel uses glycolic acid, irritant contact dermatitis is possible. Any peel can irritate your skin, especially if the concentration of chemicals is too high or you use them too often. Also, if your skin is irritated before you use a chemical peel, the chemicals may penetrate too deeply. Rarely, you may have swelling followed by skin darkening. This may happen if a superficial peel is started at a low dose and then increased steadily.

Microdermabrasion

Many physician offices and spas offer this quick, painless cosmetic treatment that does not require a doctor and has a mild effect on fine lines, wrinkles, and

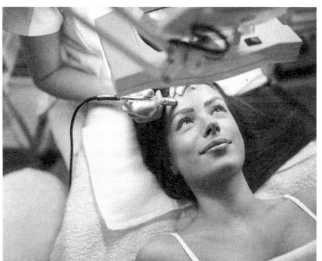

Microdermabrasion can produce moderate improvements in skin texture. In this procedure, the doctor or aesthetician abrades an area with tiny aluminum hydroxide crystals to create smoother-looking skin. No recovery time is needed.

age spots. Like a chemical peel, microdermabrasion is a physical method for superficially removing the top layers of the epidermis by lightly sanding the skin with aluminum hydroxide crystals or other similar crystals applied under high pressure; it doesn't hurt, and some people say it feels like you are being licked by a cat's sandpapery tongue. You may have some redness or swelling around the eyes, but it usually subsides the same day. Each year, about half a million microdermabrasion treatments are performed. A single treatment costs $129 on average.

Each treatment takes about 20 to 30 minutes. Typically, you'll schedule a series of six treatments, one every two weeks, and then periodic follow-up treatments to maintain the effect. Microdermabrasion treatments can be alternated with chemical peels for improved appearance.

Microneedling

This technique, performed in a doctor's office or spa, is used to treat fine lines and wrinkles. A doctor repeatedly applies an electric or battery-operated instrument (Collagen P.I.N., DermaFrac, Dermapen, Eclipse MicroPen, Juvapen, SkinPen, others) containing multiple small, thin, sharp needles to the skin to puncture it, creating tiny injuries that will stimulate the production of collagen and elastin. Therapeutic substances, such as hyaluronic acid or ascorbic acid, can be applied before or after needling so the substance penetrates deeply. The procedure takes 15 to 30 minutes on the face and feels like sandpaper rubbing against the skin; a topical anesthetic can be applied if you feel significant discomfort.

Afterward, the treated skin may look red or puffy for a couple of days. There is a small risk that the therapeutic substance might be absorbed throughout your body.

Your skin may look smoother right away, and its appearance may continue to improve for up to a year. A series of two to three treatments spaced six to eight weeks apart is typically recommended. Microneedling can be performed along with radiofrequency skin tightening (see "Radiofrequency," page 48). Microneedling instruments are also sold for home use (see "Home treatments and devices," page 48).

Laser resurfacing

Improvements in laser technology have created many options in the treatment of photoaged skin. Lasers remove moderate to deep lines and wrinkles while significantly improving skin tone, texture, and tightness. Their ability to target very specific types of cells in distinct skin layers enables them to treat conditions that were previously impossible to treat, such as port-wine stains, pigmented birthmarks, and spider veins. They can also erase acne pits and many other scars.

Lasers work by emitting intense beams of bright "light" that transfer high levels of energy to a target in or on the skin. There, the energy is converted to heat. Each laser produces a specific single wavelength, or color, of light—from the invisible infrared to visible reds, yellows, and greens. A laser's wavelength influences how deeply it penetrates the skin and how it will affect the skin. Different wavelengths work best on different problems. For example, yellow and green wavelengths target the red pigments of port-wine stains or spider veins, while infrared lasers are typically used to remove wrinkles, fine lines, and crow's feet.

Lasers also vary by the duration of their pulses. The duration of the pulse of light determines how a laser affects targeted tissue. Almost all cosmetic procedures require lasers that emit pulsed light, which

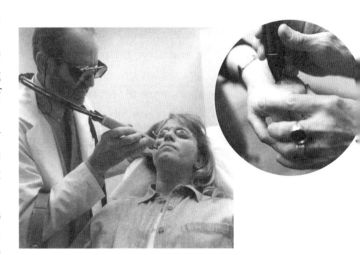

The pulsed dye laser (above left) is used to treat red spots, dilated blood vessels, spider veins, and broken capillaries. This laser emits a yellow light, which targets reddish pigments in the skin.

The Q-switched laser (above right) gives off bursts of energy that are absorbed by brown pigments in the skin. As a result, this laser is used to eliminate liver spots, freckles, and some tattoos.

confers the precise control needed to alter only the intended skin layers or pigments and leave the surrounding skin unaffected.

Most laser procedures are bloodless and can be controlled precisely, reducing the risk for injury or scarring. Recovery times for laser procedures vary depending on the laser used and the depth of treatment.

Fractional laser resurfacing

Fractional laser resurfacing has generally replaced older methods of laser resurfacing because it improves the skin's texture and appearance with a relatively short recovery time. Instead of removing the entire surface of the skin, it treats a fraction of the skin's surface. The laser produces microscopic columns of thermal damage, leaving the surrounding skin cells intact (see Figure 5). The body's natural healing process creates new, healthy tissue to replace the columns of affected tissue—improving the skin condition being treated. There are two kinds of fractional resurfacing: ablative and non-ablative. (Ablative techniques are called that because they ablate—that is, remove or destroy—the surface of the skin.) Both offer the advantage of shorter recovery time with lowered risk of scarring, changes in pigmentation, or infection compared with the older technique of non-fractional resurfacing. Because of these attributes, fractional resurfacing is also safer than other methods for people with darker skin.

Figure 5: Evolution of a laser

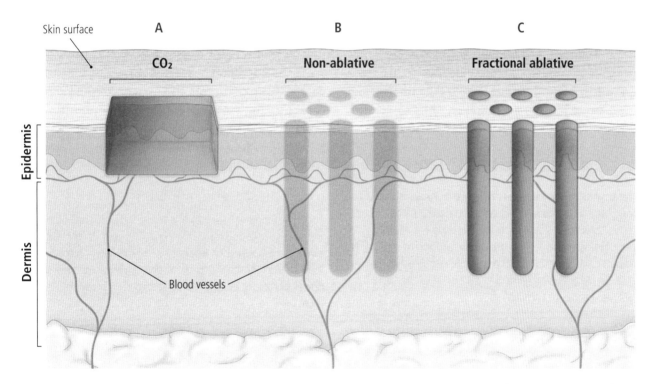

A. Introduced in the early 1990s, CO_2 laser resurfacing worked by ablating (removing) the entire surface of the skin in the treated area, reducing wrinkles and discolorations but causing extensive oozing, scabbing, and redness requiring several weeks of recovery time.

B. Next came non-ablative laser and photofacial treatments, which do not remove surface skin. These methods require little or no recovery time but are less effective at improving skin appearance. They are available in fractional versions (meaning the energy is applied in a grid of tiny dots, as shown above) and non-fractional versions.

C. Dermatologists then developed fractional ablative CO_2 and erbium:YAG laser treatments that treat skin in a grid of dots, removing tiny columns of skin while leaving most of the surface intact. This method is more effective than the non-ablative methods, with recovery time of only about 10 days.

Fractional non-ablative laser resurfacing. This procedure does not remove surface skin but rather targets deeper skin layers, which then heal by forming new collagen. Experts typically recommend four to six treatments, which are usually done four to six weeks apart. For these treatments, you will need only topical anesthesia to control pain. Some doctors also use a hand-held cool air device that chills the skin and makes the procedure more comfortable. Your skin will be red for up to a week, and you may have mild swelling for a couple of days.

You may notice some reduction of wrinkles and improvement in skin texture, pigmentation, and tightness almost immediately. Each treatment stimulates the process of new collagen formation, and results are progressive, with the best results appearing in about two to three months. Repeat treatments on a regular basis may be used to maintain the effects. The cost is roughly $500 or more for each treatment in a series. Non-ablative lasers include Clear + Brilliant, Fraxel DUAL, Fraxel re:store, and Palomar Lux 1540.

Fractional ablative laser resurfacing. This procedure destroys (ablates) targeted skin on the surface and lower levels, which is then replaced by new, healthy collagen and epidermal tissue. It can tighten skin or remove spots with a single treatment (which costs somewhere between $1,000 and $2,500 depending on the number and size of the sites being treated), although a single, higher-dose treatment requires greater healing time than multiple, lower-dose treatments. Itching and swelling last up to one week, but mild redness can persist for months. Other possible side effects include scarring, changes in skin color, or a flare-up of the herpes virus (a virus that causes cold sores) in people who carry that infection. Examples of fractional ablative lasers include Active FX, Deep FX, Fraxel re:pair SST, and SmartXide DOX.

Non-fractional ablative laser resurfacing

Once the only laser treatment for cosmetic uses, pulsed or scanned non-fractional ablative laser resurfacing is now reserved for advanced photodamage and severe acne scars. It is most effective against damage to the epidermis and superficial layers of the dermis, including lines and wrinkles from sun damage, acne scars, actinic keratosis, freckles, age spots, and dull patches caused by photodamage. It cannot remove very deep lines and wrinkles, however; for those, you

Lasers for skin discoloration, tattoo and hair removal, and more

Lasers can improve a variety of specific problems, including port-wine stains, red cheeks and noses, dilated blood vessels, spider veins, age spots, and freckles—in addition to smoothing wrinkles. They are also used for removing unwanted hair and tattoos. The type of laser selected depends on the problem, particularly the color of the spots or pigmented areas to be removed.

Red spots, dilated blood vessels, spider veins, and broken capillaries require lasers that target the red pigments in hemoglobin, a component in blood, to eliminate these imperfections. (Spider veins form when groups of blood vessels close to the surface of the skin dilate, creating a fine network of red, blue, or purple veins on the thighs, calves, and ankles.) Pulsed dye lasers, which emit a yellow light, target these reddish pigments. These lasers are also used for minimizing wrinkles and increasing collagen and elastin in the skin. Side effects include swelling for a day and sometimes bruising. Potassium titanyl phosphate (KTP) lasers, which emit green light, also treat broken capillaries. Treatments produce very mild redness or puffiness.

For brown pigment such as age spots, freckles, and some tattoos (see "Tattoo removal," page 47), your doctor will likely use a Q-switched laser or one of the newer picosecond lasers—alexandrite, Nd:YAG, or ruby—which emit very short pulses of intense energy that is absorbed by brown pigments.

Longer pulses of the same wavelength used to treat pigmented lesions destroy larger targets, and so are helpful for removing unwanted dark hair on the face or body (most commonly the chin, upper lip, armpit, bikini area, or back). To date, no laser effectively removes light or gray hairs, which lack dark pigments.

The length of time for treatment and recovery varies depending on the laser, the size of the treated area, and the extent of the problem. Your doctor can provide you with detailed information about how the procedure will be done and what you will need to do during the recovery period.

may need soft-tissue fillers (see page 40). Recovery time for ablative non-fractional resurfacing can be lengthy; potential side effects include permanently lightened skin, prolonged redness and inflammation, infection, and scarring. Other, less common complications include acne and darkened skin.

Carbon dioxide (CO2) laser resurfacing. This procedure penetrates more deeply than the erbium:YAG laser (see below). It also creates more thermal damage in the dermis, so it produces the most dramatic results in erasing deep lines and wrinkles. In addition, it can tighten the skin significantly. The intense heat of the CO_2 laser is painful, but you'll receive a local anesthetic to blunt the pain. Because this laser sometimes lightens skin, it requires extra caution when treating people with olive-colored or dark skin.

Erbium:YAG laser resurfacing. This procedure generates less heat and removes a thinner skin layer on one pass. It is therefore less painful, and recovery time is shorter. Because the erbium:YAG laser penetrates the skin only about one-fifth as deeply as the CO_2 laser, it is usually selected for treating less severe lines and wrinkles. With one or two passes, the erbium:YAG laser moderately improves severe photoaging and eliminates many wrinkles. But your doctor can also make multiple passes to achieve the same dramatic results as with the CO_2 laser.

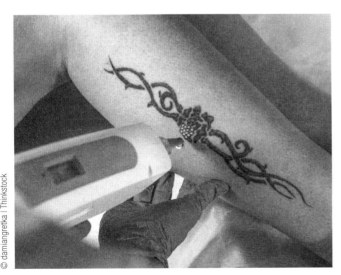

Tattoos are easy to apply, but not so easy to remove. Removal may require two or more lasers that target different colors, and the process can be painful. The doctor may inject a painkiller beforehand to ease your discomfort during the procedure.

Tattoo removal

Once considered a sign of rebellion, tattoos have become trendy in recent years. About one in four Americans, particularly those under age 40, have at least one tattoo, according to polls. But 25% of them later regret getting inked, and not surprisingly, laser tattoo removal is also on the rise. One survey found that laser tattoo removal procedures rose by 32% from 2011 to 2012.

Lasers emit intense pulses of light that mechanically break up ink particles embedded within the skin. The ink particles get absorbed and eventually eliminated through the body's waste-filtering (lymphatic) system. Compared with most cosmetic laser treatments, tattoo removal is more painful because of the heat generated when the light hits the ink. Most doctors use devices that blow cool air over the skin during treatment to lessen discomfort. If you have a large, elaborate tattoo, most doctors will inject an anesthetic to ease pain during the procedure.

The cost for each laser session ranges from $300 to $600 (average $356), and people usually need multiple sessions—the larger or more complicated the tattoo, the more sessions. Studies suggest fewer treatments are needed with the newer, picosecond alexandrite lasers (such as Picosure, Cutera Enlighten, and Candela PicoSure) than with Q-switched lasers, which were the go-to lasers for tattoo removal in the past. But tattoo removal may require at least two different lasers that target different colors. Black, blue, and red inks tend to fade more completely, while yellow, orange, and green inks are more difficult to erase. In many cases, the tattoo doesn't completely disappear. Rarely, you may notice changes in skin texture or scarring.

Combination therapy. Both types of lasers—or a single, dual-mode instrument that incorporates both—can also be used during a treatment. This approach draws on the strengths of each laser, but there still may be substantial side effects, such as scarring or pigment changes.

The cost for ablative laser resurfacing varies, but it may start around $2,100 for a portion of the face and $6,000 to $8,000 for the full face.

Skin tightening and lifting techniques

These procedures work by heating the deeper skin layers and stimulating collagen growth without damaging the skin's outer layer. The therapies use devices that emit radiofrequency, pulsed light, or ultrasound energy. Most target skin around the face and neck and require multiple treatments.

Radiofrequency

Radiofrequency treatment—sometimes called a non-surgical facelift—is used to tighten lax, sagging skin on cheeks, jowls, and brows. While it can be uncomfortable, it requires little to no recovery time, compared with two to three weeks for facelift surgery. But unlike a surgical facelift, radiofrequency doesn't lift muscle, so it's not as useful for people with advanced wrinkling and very saggy skin. It is more helpful to people in their late 30s to early 60s who have mild skin looseness and wrinkling.

The first FDA-approved radiofrequency device, Thermage, treats fine lines around the eyes, forehead wrinkles, sagging jowls and cheeks, and other areas on the body. Today, multiple devices with differing characteristics are made by several different companies; examples include Aluma, Elos, and Pellevé.

A radiofrequency device delivers an electromagnetic current to the skin, while a cooling treatment tip protects the epidermis. The doctor can control the amount of energy delivered by the device. The skin's natural resistance slows the flow of electrons, which creates an intense, uniform, and sustained heat to the tissues within the skin. The heat penetrates more deeply into the dermis and subdermal layers than lasers do in resurfacing. Treatment takes an hour or two, depending on the size of the area being treated and the number of passes the doctor makes. You can get back to your daily life immediately. You may have a little redness for an hour, but rarely any swelling, bruising, or pain. Side effects are uncommon and usually temporary.

Usually only one treatment is needed. You may see immediate improvement, but the full benefits appear gradually over four to six months as collagen production continues. Results may last for up to two years. Treating the lower face and neck costs approximately $3,000, the upper face $2,000, and the full face $4,500.

A more invasive technique for sagging neck skin can be performed with the ThermiTight device. The doctor numbs the area to be treated, makes a nick in the skin, and inserts a cannula (thin tube) into the skin to deliver the radiofrequency energy deeply into the subdermal layer. Discomfort is minimal.

Home treatments and devices

Cosmetic treatments that you can do at home are becoming increasingly common and can be bought without a prescription directly from manufacturers, from beauty stores such as Sephora and Ulta, and at other retailers. For instance, mild chemical peels (Caudalie Glycolic Peel, Dr. Dennis Gross Alpha-Beta Peel, and many others), microdermabrasion kits (PMD Personal Microderm devices, Silk'n ReVit Diamond Microdermabrasion System), and devices for skin care and hair removal are available for self-use. The chemical peels and microdermabrasion kits use the same ingredients as professionals do, but in lower concentrations. They can remove dead skin and diminish scars and fine lines, safely and conveniently, for a fraction of the cost of professional treatment. But the results are less dramatic. They work best for minor skin flaws.

Home laser, LED light, electrocurrent, and ultrasound treatments are also less powerful than physician- and aesthetician-delivered therapy, but they can be effective if you have the patience to perform treatments on a frequent basis for many weeks or months. They can also be used to maintain the effects of office treatments. Brand names include Lux Renew (ultrasound plus LED lights); Ziip (an electrical current device); Baby Quasar Clear Rayz, LightStim for Acne, Skin Inc. Optimizer Voyage Tri-Light, and Silk'n Face FX (LED light devices); and Tria Age-Defying Laser (laser to treat fine lines). Be sure to read and follow directions for these products to use them safely.

Laser hair removal devices (No!No!, Tria) can be used to permanently remove unwanted black or brown body hair. These devices are not recommended for people who are tan, have darker skin, or have a skin condition. More recent arrivals on the market are intense pulsed light devices (the Gillette Venus Silk-Expert Powered by Braun and the Silk'n hair removal device) to reduce unwanted hair growth.

There are also a variety of home microneedling rollers (Dermaroller, Drs. Rodan and Fields, Skin Medix) that can be used to deliver retinols, moisturizers, and other compounds deeply into the skin. It's important to sterilize these rollers with an alcohol bath after every use to prevent infections.

Fractional high-intensity focused radiofrequency

New instruments (Endymed Intensif, Infini) have recently been introduced that combine both radiofrequency and microneedling (see page 44). The microneedling punctures the skin and allows the radiofrequency energy to be delivered within the skin to tighten it up by stimulating collagen and elastin production. Discomfort is minimal, and the technique works well for tightening skin on the neck and face. Three treatments are typically needed, at a cost of around $2,000 each.

Ultrasound therapy

Focused or intense ultrasound therapy works to tighten skin by causing molecules under the skin to vibrate, creating the heat that stimulates collagen formation. The ultrasound device (called the Ulthera System) is similar to an ultrasound used to create pictures of a developing baby, although it only penetrates about 8 millimeters beneath the skin. But this enables the clinician to target the treatment more precisely.

Each treatment takes about 60 to 90 minutes. Most people just have one treatment, but some benefit from additional sessions. The results appear gradually over two to three months, and sometimes up to six months. Side effects include discomfort during the treatment, redness that usually goes away within a few hours, and swelling that may last a few days. The treated area may also be tender or tingle when touched for several weeks. A full face and neck treatment costs about $3,000. Treating just the brow area is about $350.

Light-based therapy

These treatments use low-level light (as opposed to the intense light of a laser) to stimulate the skin's production of collagen. They are best for addressing mild to moderate skin discolorations and imperfections.

Pulsed light therapy

Sometimes referred to as a "photo facial," pulsed light therapy (Cutera Xeo, Icon, others) can improve mild to moderate photodamage to skin color and texture with no recovery time and few complications. In addition to improving the skin's texture and tone, pulsed light therapy can diminish freckles, red spots, age spots, and dilated blood vessels. It may also be used to treat unwanted dark hair and the red cheeks or nose seen with rosacea. This treatment uses an intense pulsed light (IPL) device. It's not a laser; it emits bursts of broadband light energy that penetrates the epidermis and dermis and promotes new collagen growth. IPL treatment does not need to be performed in a doctor's office and is often offered in salons and spas.

For the procedure, the practitioner will coat your face with a gel and cover your eyes to protect them from the pulse of light. When the device flashes, you'll feel a quick zap of heat, like the snap of a rubber band. Each flash treats an area about the size of a quarter, and you may have two or three passes in a 30- to 60-minute session. Afterward, you may have some redness or blotchiness for a day or two.

Most practitioners recommend four to six sessions, each costing approximately $350, spaced three or four weeks apart. Improvement is gradual, with most people able to notice a difference after three treatments. Maintenance treatments are required a few times a year. Side effects can include sunburn, loss or increase of skin pigmentation, and scarring.

Photodynamic therapy

In addition to removing actinic keratosis (see "Treating actinic keratosis," page 20), photodynamic therapy is used to reduce fine lines and blotchiness from photoaging, as well as to rejuvenate the entire face and treat acne. Each treatment takes 45 to 90 minutes, and one to six treatments may be needed, with a cost of about $800 per treatment. Photodynamic therapy is best done by a doctor.

LED photomodulation

LED photomodulation, which uses light produced by light-emitting diodes, is a reasonably effective way to induce subtle improvements in the skin for people with mild to moderate sun damage. Photomodulation, which is painless, doesn't damage the surface or deeper layers of skin. Instead, it signals cells that remodel the collagen in the dermis. During this procedure, your face will be exposed to continuous or pulsed yellow (known as Gentle Waves) or red (ProLight Red/Infrared) LED light for 30 seconds to three minutes. Photomodulation can complement almost any other procedure on your face and works on all skin types. It can also rapidly treat a large area in one brief session, with no aftereffects. Its effects may be subtle, however, and eight to 10 treatments are usually required, with ongoing treatments needed to maintain the results.

In addition to improving sun damage, LED photomodulation can be used to help speed healing following other laser treatments. The treatment can be done by a doctor, nurse, or medical assistant.

If you're undecided …

Are cosmetic treatments worth the time, money, and potential side effects? Only you can answer that question. But as these treatments improve, they have in some ways become like sunscreen or topical retinoids, in that some people, especially women, have come to rely on semi-regular treatments to help prevent the appearance of aging skin and leave them looking younger and healthier.

For some, the payoff is a sense of better competitiveness in the job market. For others, it's enhanced self-esteem. In fact, some research postulates that aesthetic procedures—especially botulinum toxin—may lead to unconscious changes in your muscle movement and even your mood. According to doctors, people who have cosmetic procedures often report that people respond to them differently afterward, saying things like "You used to look so angry!"

But remember, these are procedures with substantial price tags and potential side effects. The decision to alter your appearance is an important one that should be done in consultation with a doctor who understands and respects your wishes. Be sure you understand all the costs involved, the total time commitment (including recovery), as well as how long the treatment's effects are likely to last and any possible side effects you may experience.

And be realistic. You cannot achieve perfection—only improvement. ◗

Resources

Organizations

American Academy of Cosmetic Surgery
225 W. Wacker Drive, Suite 650
Chicago, IL 60606
312-981-6760
www.cosmeticsurgery.org

Represents surgeons who work in postgraduate medical education in cosmetic surgery. Sponsors a surgeon referral service. The website contains a "For Patients" information channel.

American Academy of Dermatology
P.O. Box 4014
Schaumburg, IL 60168
888-462-3372 (toll-free)
www.aad.org

The largest of all dermatologic associations. The website provides information on the diagnosis and medical, surgical, and cosmetic treatment of conditions of the skin, hair, and nails, and a "Find a Dermatologist" tool.

American Academy of Facial Plastic and Reconstructive Surgery
310 S. Henry St.
Alexandria, VA 22314
703-299-9291
www.aafprs.org

An association of plastic and reconstructive surgeons who focus on surgery of the face, head, and neck. Sponsors programs of free care for those with deformities from congenital conditions and trauma, including domestic violence and war.

American Board of Medical Specialties
353 N. Clark St.
Chicago, IL 60654
312-436-2600
866-275-2267 (toll-free physician verification)
www.abms.org

Operates a phone and online service to help members of the public verify the board-certification status of physicians.

American Society for Aesthetic Plastic Surgery
11262 Monarch St.
Garden Grove, CA 92841
800-364-2147 (toll-free)
www.surgery.org

The leading organization of cosmetic plastic surgeons. The website offers patient education about a wide range of procedures and a surgeon finder service. There is also an "Ask a Plastic Surgeon" feature and cost information.

American Society for Dermatologic Surgery
5550 Meadowbrook Drive, Suite 120
Rolling Meadows, IL 60008
847-956-0900
www.asds.net

Provides information on its website regarding the subspecialty of dermatologic surgery and offers referrals to board-certified dermatologic surgeons.

American Society for Laser Medicine and Surgery
2100 Stewart Ave., Suite 240
Wausau, WI 54401
877-258-6028 (toll-free)
www.aslms.org

Promotes research, safety, and quality standards in the field of laser medicine. The website offers an online doctor referral service as well as information on new procedures in laser medicine.

American Society of Plastic Surgeons
444 E. Algonquin Road
Arlington Heights, IL 60005
847-228-9900
www.plasticsurgery.org

Represents surgeons certified by the American Board of Plastic Surgery or the Royal College of Physicians and Surgeons of Canada. The website offers information on a variety of procedures and a surgeon referral service.

FDA Cosmetics
www.fda.gov/cosmetics

Informational website for consumers interested in the safety and effectiveness of cosmetics ingredients, as well as the regulation of cosmetics.

National Psoriasis Foundation
6600 S.W. 92nd Ave., Suite 300
Portland, OR 97223
800-723-9166 (toll-free)
www.psoriasis.org

Provides educational materials on the causes, diagnosis, and treatment of psoriasis. The website also includes patient forums, free advice services, and referrals to expert health professionals and clinical trials.

Skin Cancer Foundation
149 Madison Ave., Suite 901
New York, NY 10016
212-725-5176
www.skincancer.org

Seeks to educate the public on the prevention, detection, and treatment of skin cancer. The website contains useful information on actinic keratosis, basal and squamous cell carcinomas, and melanoma, as well as advice on prevention.

Glossary

actinic keratosis: Scaly pink or red-brown raised spots or patches caused by overexposure to the sun. Actinic keratosis may be a precursor to skin cancer.

aesthetician: Licensed skin care professional who performs such procedures as deep cleansing, low-grade chemical peels, microdermabrasion, and postsurgical skin care.

alpha hydroxy acids: Fruit-derived acids used in creams and lotions to act as exfoliants.

autologous fat transplant: Removal of fat from one part of the body to use as filler in another part, for example, to fill wrinkles and lines in the face and lips.

basal cell carcinoma: The most common skin cancer. Basal cell carcinoma doesn't spread to internal organs.

botulinum toxin A: A substance that eases the appearance of some facial wrinkles by inhibiting chemical messengers (neurotransmitters) that cause muscles to contract.

chemical peel: Use of mild to caustic chemical solutions to wound the outer layer of the epidermis and encourage new collagen growth.

collagen: A fibrous protein that's the main component of connective tissue.

contact dermatitis: A rash or irritation that occurs when a person's skin comes into contact with an offending substance.

dermis: The middle layer of skin, which contains blood and lymph vessels, nerves, hair follicles, and glands that produce sweat and oil.

elastin: The protein that gives skin its elasticity.

epidermis: The outermost layer of skin.

humectant: An agent used in moisturizers; binds water to the skin to promote hydration.

intense pulsed light (IPL): White light that's used in skin-resurfacing procedures and hair removal.

keratinocytes: Cells of the epidermis that produce a tough protein called keratin and form a soft, protective sheet for the body.

Langerhans cells: Cells in the outermost layer of skin, the epidermis, that form the front-line defenses of the immune system. Discovered by German physician Paul Langerhans.

laser: The acronym of "light amplification by the stimulated emission of radiation." Lasers produce intense beams of light that generate heat used in surgery, removal of pigmented lesions, and skin rejuvenation.

melanocytes: Cells deep in the epidermis that produce melanin, the skin's pigment.

melanoma: The most serious type of skin cancer, originating in the pigment-producing cells known as melanocytes.

melomental folds: Creases that run from the corners of the mouth to the chin; sometimes called marionette lines.

nasolabial folds: Creases that run from each side of the nose to the corners of the mouth; sometimes called smile lines.

photodynamic therapy: A treatment for actinic keratosis that uses light exposure to activate a therapeutic agent.

skin resurfacing: Any of several approaches to improve skin texture, tone, wrinkle appearance, and discolorations by promoting new collagen and epidermal growth. Chemical peels, dermabrasion, microdermabrasion, and laser procedures are skin-resurfacing techniques.

squamous cell carcinoma: A common skin cancer, rarely fatal, that can spread to the lymph nodes and internal organs.

subcutaneous tissue: The deepest layer of skin, consisting of connective tissue and fat.